From Crib to
 Kindergarten

From Crib to Kindergarten

The Essential Child Safety Guide

Dorothy A. Drago, M.P.H.

THE JOHNS HOPKINS UNIVERSITY PRESS
Baltimore

Note to readers

This book provides information to help parents and other caregivers keep children safe from injury. The information in this book is as reliable and as up-to-date as possible, but neither the author nor the publisher bears responsibility for the safety of an individual child. That responsibility lies with the person providing care for the child.

This book is not intended to provide medical or legal advice. The services of a competent professional should be obtained whenever medical, legal, or other specific advice is needed. The publisher and the author make no warranty, either express or implied, regarding the recommendations offered or the practices described; nor does the publisher or the author assume liability for any consequences arising from the use of the content of this book.

© 2007 The Johns Hopkins University Press
All rights reserved. Published 2007
Printed in the United States of America on acid-free paper
9 8 7 6 5 4 3 2 1

The Johns Hopkins University Press
2715 North Charles Street
Baltimore, Maryland 21218-4363
www.press.jhu.edu

Library of Congress Cataloging-in-Publication Data

Drago, Dorothy A., 1946–
    From crib to kindergarten : the essential child safety guide / Dorothy A. Drago.
        p. cm.
    Includes bibliographical references and index.
    ISBN-13: 978-0-8018-8569-3 (hardcover : alk. paper)
    ISBN-13: 978-0-8018-8570-9 (pbk. : alk. paper)
    ISBN-10: 0-8018-8569-8 (hardcover : alk. paper)
    ISBN-10: 0-8018-8570-1 (pbk. : alk. paper)
    1. Children's accidents—Prevention. 2. Pediatric emergencies—Prevention.
3. Safety education. I. Title.
RJ370.D73 2007
613.6′083—dc22
                                                          2006020809

A catalog record for this book is available from the British Library.

Illustrations on pages 32, 59, 60, 61, 63 (top), 73, 91, 94, 127, and 154 are by Jacqueline Schaffer. Illustrations on pages 81 and 139 are from the U.S. Consumer Product Safety Commission and are reproduced with permission of ASTM International; the others are in the public domain. Illustrations on page 86 are used with permission of Fisher-Price, Inc., East Aurora, New York 14052; Fisher-Price notes: "There are many types of retention systems on helmets, and it is very important to read and understand the fit instructions and warnings contained in the manual that came with the helmet." All other illustrations are by Loel Barr.

Contents

Preface

You are almost certainly reading this book because you have children in your life who mean the world to you. Your children or grandchildren or nieces or nephews or next-door neighbors light up the lives of everyone they touch, and you want to keep those precious children safe from all harm.

As an injury prevention specialist, I, too, care very deeply about keeping children safe. I study injury trends, identify the causes of injuries, and recommend ways to prevent injury. I wrote this book to give you the benefit of my work and my experience.

Before I describe what this book is about and how it is organized, let me say a few words about what it is *not*. Above all, this is not a book meant to instill fear or anxiety. By helping you understand how to keep your child safe, I hope to make you feel more confident as you and your child go about your daily lives. Nor is this a book about childhood development, although it does touch on developmental milestones to explain how and why children are at risk for different injuries at different developmental stages. Finally, this is not a guide to buying specific products, although it does discuss hazards, regulations, and labeling information for most of the kinds of products used around babies and children. *This is a book that will help you recognize and reduce hazards so that your children can be as safe from injury as possible.*

Injury can be defined simply as physical damage to the body. In the past, the word *accident* was used to describe an event that resulted in injury, but over time the scientific study of injury has revealed that there are underlying factors that can predict injury, and thus it has become clear that injuries are not random or chance events, as the word *accident* suggests. Now we use the term *unintentional injury*. It is unsettling at the least to realize that unintentional injury is the leading cause of death among children. Happily, the study of injury has also revealed that steps can be taken to prevent or minimize injury.

A hazard can also be defined simply as any condition that has the potential to cause injury. Recognizing hazards (called "hazard identification"), like any other skill, requires education, training, and experience. In reading this book, you are educating yourself in how to identify hazards and eliminate them. As you gain experience in identifying and eliminating hazards, you will reap the huge benefit of providing a safer environment for your child.

Children aged newborn to five years old spend most of their time at home, and they are most likely to be injured in and around the home. That's why this book focuses on young children within the home setting. One purpose of this book is to communicate the message that children are vulnerable to different injuries at different ages. The changes in children's vulnerability to injury are related to changes in their size, shape, physical and cognitive abilities, and behavior patterns.

Another purpose of this book is to provide specific information about how to reduce hazards and create a safer home environment for your children. To that end, each chapter

- explains and illustrates injury patterns and describes when children are at risk for these injuries;
- lists key prevention methods; and concludes with
- a safety checklist.

Charts that summarize key injury prevention information from each chapter can be found in the appendix at the end of the text. The checklists and summary charts provide quick access to key information that is relevant for your child's age.

Throughout this book, you will see illustrations that are labeled with a special symbol—a triangle containing an exclamation point. This symbol means, "Watch out! This is not safe!"

In the first chapter, I provide more information about injury and injury prevention and begin to describe why children are at risk for specific injuries at specific ages. The core of the book is organized by the daily routines in a child's life: sleeping, bathing and dressing, eating, playing, and travel. Again, in describing the hazards in these routines I do not mean to scare readers but rather to help readers reduce or eliminate the hazards (which, as noted, have the potential to cause serious injury and death). The last two chapters focus on the physical household environment, from the backyard to the family room, to help you recognize the hazards all around the home. Following the appendix of charts is a list of useful resources you may want to consult to keep current on safety issues.

I encourage you to use this book as a resource and reference guide throughout the first five years of your child's life, referring to specific sections as often as you need to. Use the charts and checklists as quick reminders of when (at what age) children are at greatest risk for certain injuries, and for reminders about key prevention measures you can take. Share your knowledge with anyone who is involved in your children's care, from sitters and other caregivers to grandparents and others.

What I want more than anything is for this book to help you keep your children as injury free as possible through their first five years of life.

From Crib to
Kindergarten

1

❦ Keeping Your Child Safe from Injury

An Introduction

The Myths and Realities of Childhood Injury

Many people have beliefs about how injuries occur and how they can be prevented. Often, however, these beliefs reflect myths rather than reality. One common myth is that an injury is a random event—the result of chance, bad luck, or something else over which we have no control. This myth has had a long life, in part because the word *accident* perpetuates the notion that injuries occur in unpredictable ways. Today, injury prevention specialists have replaced *accident* with *unintentional injury*. Injuries are either intentional (the result of a deliberate act, such as abuse or violence) or unintentional (the result of a person's interacting with a product or condition in a particular environment). The reality is this: we *can* predict and, therefore, *can* prevent unintentional injury.

Another myth is that injury prevention is just a matter of common sense. Although common sense can help prevent injuries, effective injury prevention strategies are based on scientific principles. Many disciplines are involved in injury prevention, including epidemiology, hazard analysis, human factors analysis, engineering, biology, physics, biomechanics, and communication science.

Think of an unintentional injury as an event that occurs on a timeline. That is, some scenario—events, personal characteristics, products, or environmental conditions—sets the stage for an injury to be possible. If these events, characteristics, or conditions interact in a certain way, a predictable injury could occur. Once an injury has occurred, further events are set in motion. For example, a bystander reacts, someone calls 911, or someone rescues the injured person from more serious injury.

Here's an example of a timeline of an unintentional injury:

On a warm day, a backyard above-ground swimming pool has just been used by a family taking a swim before lunch. The pool does not have a pool cover. The family consists of a mother, a father, and three children, aged eight, five, and two years. The eight-year-old is the last one to leave the pool area. His hands are full—he is carrying shoes, towels, and goggles—so he can't get a good grip on the gate when he closes it. As a result the latch does not lock, and the gate stays ajar.

Inside the house, the father prepares lunch while the mother gets the two-year-old into dry clothes. The older children take care of themselves and play a video game in the den until lunch is ready. The mother sends her youngest child into the den with one of his toys, telling the older children to keep an eye on him while she takes a quick shower. The older children, however, get involved in their game and do not realize that their brother has left the den and headed for the pool.

When the mother gets out of the shower and goes to check on the children, she realizes the youngster is missing. Her instinct is to call for him and hurry to the pool. She sees him floating face down and immediately pulls him out of the water and begins CPR. The father, alerted to what has happened, calls 911. Paramedics arrive in two minutes and take over the mother's efforts.

This child is fortunate and survives because he was found in time and because his mother knew CPR.

You can see that pre-injury events—those that set the stage for an injury—may unfold over time, but the injury itself happens in an instant. The outcome of the injury depends on how quickly rescue efforts begin and how effective they are.

You can also see that even though the stage had been set for an injury, if the two-year-old boy had not gone outside, he would not have almost drowned. Or had he gone outside but found the pool gate locked, he would not have ended up in the pool. Changing even one aspect of the scenario leads to a different outcome.

Here's another example:

A grandmother visits her daughter and two-year-old grandson for the weekend. The grandmother takes blood pressure medication and keeps it in her purse when she travels. For convenience, she has transferred a weekend's worth of medication from its child-resistant package to a pillbox with a simple lid.

When she arrives at her daughter's home and settles into the guest room, she sets her purse on the bed. Later on, she comes across her grandson looking in her purse. She sees that the pillbox has been opened and is empty.

The boy's mother calls a poison hotline. Based on the type of medication, she is instructed to take her son to the local emergency department. There the medical staff monitor and treat him, and he is released the next morning.

From both of these examples, you can appreciate why we prefer injury prevention efforts—those that interrupt the pre-injury scenario so that an injury never occurs—to injury control efforts, those that help minimize the consequences of an injury once it has occurred. But because it is not always possible to prevent injury, it is also important to control injury. In both of the scenarios above, the injury prevention effort (the locking gate and the child-resistant cap) failed because of human error. In both cases, the injury control effort worked, because the injury was reversed by immediate and appropriate actions (CPR and emergency department treatment).

Human error is not a negative term. We all make mistakes: we all get fatigued, stressed, distracted, or confused at times, or we fail to communicate with each other, and any of these conditions can lead to our making mistakes. Good injury prevention solutions always consider human factors, including what a person may do wrong and what the consequences could be.

What Defines an Injury?

People recognize an injury when they see one—a cut, a scrape, blood, swelling, redness, loss of consciousness, and so on. People may even recognize an injury when visual clues are missing, for example when someone has experienced hearing damage, hyperthermia (excessive heat), or a closed head injury (a blow to the head that doesn't break the skin). But what's the underlying cause—the biological basis—of injury? Put simply, injury results when the body's tolerance to absorb energy is exceeded.

Intuitively, you know that energy is associated with moving objects, like a car, a train, or a thrown baseball, and that if a person were struck by any of these objects, the energy in the moving object would be greater than the body's ability to absorb it without injury. The energy associated with moving objects or physical force is called kinetic or mechanical energy. Other kinds of energy are thermal (related to temperature), electrical (related to electric current), chemical (related to chemical substances and drugs), and radiation (related to changes in atomic structure; examples are the production of radon gas and x-rays). All of these five types of energy can cause injury. Another cause of injury is an absence of or interference with life requirements—something a person needs to live, such as oxygen. Examples of these injuries include drowning and suffocation.

There are only six possible causes of injury, then: five kinds of energy and the lack of a life requirement. The potential for injury from any of these types of energy or from lacking a life requirement is called a *hazard*. So there are mechanical hazards, thermal hazards, electrical hazards, chemical hazards, radiation hazards, and hazards that remove or interrupt life requirements. A classic approach to injury prevention is to identify hazards associated with a product or an activity and eliminate or reduce those hazards. Removing a hazard is a great way to prevent injuries.

Mechanical hazards have to do with the potential for injury from physical forces, like pushing, pulling, compressing, obstructing, twisting, falling, and colliding. Here are examples of injuries from mechanical hazards:

cuts, bruises, and abrasions
broken bones
traumatic amputation
choking
foreign objects in the eye, ear, or nose

Thermal hazards have to do with temperature, either hot or cold. Injuries from thermal hazards include the following:

burns from contact with hot surfaces or open flames
scalds from contact with hot liquids or steam
hypothermia from exposure to excessive cold (a child who falls
    through thin ice while skating can suffer hypothermia)
hyperthermia from exposure to excessive heat (a child left in a
    closed vehicle on a hot day can suffer hyperthermia)

Electrical hazards have to do with electric current. Examples of injuries from electrical hazards include shocks and burns from contacting "live" wires (a child who sticks a key into an electrical outlet will receive a shock or jolt of electricity through his body). Lightning is natural electricity and is also an electrical hazard, though your chance of being struck by lightning is small.

Chemical hazards have to do with chemical substances in their solid, liquid, or gaseous states. For the focus of this book, chemical substances include medicines and pharmaceuticals, household cleaning agents, batteries, toxic gases, heavy metals (like lead, arsenic, and chromium), and automotive products (like antifreeze and motor oil). These are examples of injuries from chemical hazards:

poisoning
respiratory distress
chemical burns

Radiation hazards have to do with changes in molecular structure that result in the emission of heat or light. Most commonly, we associate exposure to radiation with long-term illness, such as leukemia, rather than with acute, or short-term, injury. You are unlikely to encounter a radiation hazard in your home that will result in acute injury.

Hazards that remove or interrupt life requirements have to do with the cutting off of a person's oxygen supply. Such hazards may cause injuries such as these:

suffocating
drowning
breathing air with insufficient oxygen (for example, the air in a house fire)

What Determines Whether an Injury Will Occur?

You interact with energy and hazards every day. Every time you cook, you are exposed to a thermal hazard and the potential for a burn, but only rarely do you get burned. When you do get burned, it might be a minor burn that you treat at home or a severe burn that requires a doctor's treatment. Whether an injury occurs depends on two things:

1. The amount of energy. Was it a warm cookie sheet or a hot cookie sheet that had just come out of a 400° F oven?
2. The ability of the body, or body part, to absorb that energy. Did you touch the hot pan with one finger, or did your toddler put his hand on the pan?

The energy can be delivered in a single exposure, like touching the hot cookie sheet, or over a number of exposures, for example eating lead-based paint chips every day for a month.

The ability of the body or body part to absorb the energy has to do with

- composition of the affected area: is it muscle, fat, bone, or an internal organ?
- size of the affected area: is it a fingertip, a hand, or an arm?
- biological maturity of the affected area: is it newly formed skin, a developing organ, or a mature bone structure?

The severity of an injury depends on the balance between the energy delivered and the energy one's body is able to safely absorb. To gain a sense of the relative severity of injuries, consider the following comparisons:

- injury from being hit by a toy car pushed along the floor *versus* injury from being hit by a real car traveling on a road at 40 mph
- injury from spilling a cup of hot soup *versus* injury from spilling a pot of boiling pasta
- injury from touching a household outlet wire *versus* injury from touching a high-voltage wire
- injury from drinking acetic acid (vinegar) *versus* injury from drinking sulfuric acid
- injury from a routine x-ray *versus* injury from an atomic bomb

Different parts of the body have different abilities to absorb energy, as illustrated by the severity of injury we would expect in the following situations:

- being struck by a hard ball in the eye as opposed to the thigh
- spilling hot tea on the fingers as opposed to the lap
- splashing drain cleaner on the forearm as opposed to drinking it
- an adult's taking five baby aspirins by mistake as opposed to a baby's being given five adult aspirins by mistake

From these examples, you can see that there is a broad range of injury possibilities, from no or minor injury at one extreme to death at the other. You also get a sense of how many variables come into play in determining if an injury will occur.

Injury prevention professionals study all the factors associated with an injury, including the person, the product, and the environment, to identify what can be changed to prevent or minimize the injury. The first choice is for the manufacturer to change the product, ideally in a way that does not require the person to do anything. We call this a passive intervention. If changing the product is not possible, another choice is to change the environment. An example of this would be to install a fence around a swimming pool. A third choice is to change the person's behavior, such as getting her to wear a bike helmet on a regular basis. This last choice is usually the least preferred, however, because it's quite difficult to change behavior, regardless of whether the person is a child or an adult.

A Brief History of Product Safety

We all use numerous consumer products in our daily lives, and we don't often give a lot of thought to the risks of their use. Today's consumer products are, on the whole, safe for their intended use, thanks to stringent safety measures. These safety measures haven't always been in place, however. The 1970s became a turning point for consumer product safety when Congress determined three things: (1) in the U.S. marketplace, there was an unacceptable number of consumer products that posed unreasonable risks of injury; (2) consumers were not able to anticipate the risks of using those products; and (3) the public needed to be protected. In 1972, therefore, Congress passed the Consumer Product Safety Act, which created the U.S. Consumer Product Safety Commission, an independent federal regulatory agency. The Commission was directed to collect injury data and investigate the causes and prevention of consumer product–related injuries, illnesses, and deaths. The Commission was given the authority to make rules and regulations, test products, recall or ban products, and impose civil and criminal penalties. The Commission was also given the responsibility to carry out some preexisting regulations, including the Flammable Fabrics Act (passed in 1953), the Refrigerator Safety Act (1956), the Federal Hazardous Substances Act (1960), and the Poison Prevention Packaging Act (1970).

Some of the earliest mandatory regulations the Commission put in place were for children's products, including cribs (effective in 1973), pacifiers (1977), rattles (1978), and small parts (1978). If you are thinking, "When I was a kid we didn't have all this protection, and I survived just fine," and if you are wondering why regulations are necessary at all, consider that many children *did* get injured or die when you were a child. Those injuries and deaths were never systematically reported or studied before the 1970s. The absence of regulatory protection was really a reflection of how little we knew about injury. The facts about injuries to children are disturbing.

Before the crib regulation, many infants died when they became trapped between slats or between a crib's side rail and mattress. Among other things, the regulation mandated that the spacing between crib slats be no greater than 2⅜ inches—this space is narrow enough to prevent an infant's being trapped between slats. The crib regulation forbade the use of wood screws, because they loosen over time and lead to gaps in a crib's frame in which an infant can become trapped. Later amendments to the crib regulation forbade dangerous cutouts in headboards and footboards, for these had been the cause of serious head- and neck-trapping incidents. Also, a voluntary standard among crib manufacturers did away with tall corner posts, which had created a strangling hazard, because clothing and cord loops were easily hooked over them or became caught on them, especially as children tried to climb out of the crib.

Before the pacifier regulation, infants and young children had choked on pacifiers that fit entirely into the mouth, and they were hanged by pacifier cords that caught on other items, like crib corner posts. Among other things, the regulation mandated that pacifier shields be large enough not to fit inside the mouth and that pacifiers not be sold with ribbons or other strings attached.

Before the rattle regulation, infants choked when rattles reached the back of the mouth and blocked the airway. One provision of the regulation was that a rattle not be smaller than a certain size to prevent this type of choking.

Before the small parts regulation, children choked on the small parts of toys. The regulation required that parts in toys and products intended for children younger than three years be too large to cause choking.

Some of the Consumer Product Safety Commission's more recent regulations have been for child-resistant cigarette lighters (effective in 1993), child-resistant multipurpose lighters (1999), bike helmets (1999) (bicycles have been regulated since 1978), and child-resistant baby oil packaging (2002). The Commission has also banned certain products for children younger than three years. These banned products include lawn darts, infant cushions, small balls, and dive sticks (hard plastic toys about seven inches long that children throw into the

and to be more severely injured than children without the disorder.

Understanding Childhood Risk Factors for Injury

At some point in life everyone will suffer some kind of unintentional injury, be it minor or serious, but children, especially those younger than five years, are at greater risk. Not only are infants and young children at greater risk overall, but their vulnerability to particular kinds of injury varies markedly at different ages from newborn to age five. For example, children older than one year rarely suffocate, while children older than four years rarely choke. Why should children of different ages be more or less likely to be injured in particular ways? The answer is that risk of injury is related to the child's abilities and limitations, which in turn are related to the child's age and stage of growth, development, and behavior.

Children go through dramatic changes in growth, development, and behavior, especially during their early years, and these changes tend to be age related. *Growth* refers to changes in a child's physical size. *Development* refers to changes in a child's maturity, including maturity of motor skills, biological (organ) systems, and intellectual abilities. *Behavior* refers to how children act and respond to different situations. In general, growth and development increase or mature with age; for example, children grow taller and master coordinated hand movements over time. Behaviors, such as mouthing (putting objects into the mouth) and throwing temper tantrums, tend to be age specific—they appear and later disappear.

A child's stage of growth, development, and behavior affects her risk of injury. An eighteen-month-old child who stands, walks, and has reasonable manual skills can reach for the medicine left in an open bottle on a bedside table. Because a child of this age tends to put everything she can into her mouth, she does exactly this with the colored pieces in the bottle, and she swallows several pills. Her organ system, however, is immature, and the medicine is toxic, so she is poisoned. When the same eighteen-month-old child falls asleep on the couch with you, she rolls away from the soft pillows, so she will not suffocate. Now consider these two scenarios for a three-month-old infant. The three-month-old who falls asleep on the couch with you cannot roll away from an obstruction, such as pillows, and may suffocate.

However, that same infant has not developed the motor skills necessary to reach bedside medicine and be poisoned by swallowing pills.

How Does Children's Growth Affect Their Injury Risk?

Changes in physical size are apparent throughout childhood. Children gain weight and grow tall at a fast pace—seemingly too fast at times! Overall, though, children are small compared with adults. Being small equates to easier access to some hazards and greater potential for injury.

Their small size can allow children to fit either partially or completely into spaces too tiny for adults. As a result, children have become trapped in spaces like toy chests, buckets, and openings in play equipment. Children have suffocated in car trunks and discarded refrigerators. They have been cut, shocked, or otherwise injured when body parts, particularly fingers, have entered spaces and contacted moving parts or electrical components.

Once they have contact with a hazard, young children are likely to suffer greater injury than adults exposed to the same hazard. A more serious injury occurs because the hazard affects a relatively larger area of a child's body. If an adult spilled a mug of hot coffee from the table, his foot and lower leg would most likely be scalded, but if an infant pulled down a mug of hot coffee from the table, her head, shoulders, chest, lower torso, and possibly buttocks and legs could be scalded. As another example, an adult might suffer traumatic amputation of his finger by contacting rotating blades, but a child may lose her entire hand.

Of course, a small size also means a small reach, so it is easy to store or place a hazardous item out of a young child's reach. Here are some easy ways to keep dangerous items away from children.

- When storing lighters, choose higher shelves over lower shelves.
- When cooking, choose back burners over front burners.
- When using small kitchen appliances, don't let the electrical cords dangle over the edge of the counter.
- When laying out the nursery, place the crib away from the window.

Children have a disproportionately large head compared with the rest of their body, and this also puts them at greater risk of injury. With a large head, most of a child's weight is concentrated high in

Newborn babies act primarily on their reflexes. At about the age of three months, they begin to gain some voluntary control of their actions. At first, they use their entire arm to reach toward objects; later, they use their entire hand to grasp objects. During the fourth and fifth months, infants progress from these large, waving motions to more skilled movements of the hands and fingers. By the sixth month, infants can hold and manipulate items. During the seventh to ninth months, infants delight in banging and throwing items and practice grasping with the thumb and forefinger (known as the pincer grasp). In later months, infants continue to practice their fine motor skills with deliberate play, like tower building, and with repetitive play, like placing lids on and off containers. Over time, their arm, hand, and finger movements become more and more refined.

Even as they develop and practice their fine motor skills, infants still find it difficult, and sometimes are completely unable, to get out of certain situations. For example, it is difficult for infants to push away items that are covering their face, like blankets or toys, which could be suffocation hazards. Infants can't remove an item from their mouth to avoid choking on it, nor can they untangle their limbs or body from loose ribbons or ties. The good news is that the limitations of their fine motor skills prevent infants from undoing child-safety locks and gates and keep them from gaining access to poisons, medicines, and other hazards.

By the end of their second year, children are able to twist, turn, hold, and manipulate objects. They scribble, turn the pages of a book, and have mastered grasping and releasing. At this age, they are also more "in" their environment, so they are manually interacting with many items, not just those intended for them. Because mental development does not progress at the same pace as fine motor skills, children of this age cannot understand the consequences of touching a hot surface or picking up a knife.

While infants and children have been developing these fine motor skills, they have also been developing gross motor skills (big movements), allowing them to roll, rock, scoot, sit, crawl, and walk. In the early months, infants have limited ability to move. During the third and fourth months, infants learn to hold up their head and chest for brief moments while lying on their tummy. They begin to rock and roll from side to side, but they don't actually move. When they reach about five months, infants can turn over by themselves. It takes nearly six months until infants begin supporting their head by the neck mus-

the body. The midpoint of a child's body weight (known as the center of gravity) is at about the level of the upper chest. An adult's center of gravity is lower, near the navel. A toddler has to bend over only a little bit before his weight shifts forward and he falls, whereas an adult can bend over much farther before being at risk of falling. In addition to their high center of gravity, toddlers are just learning about balance. This combination of factors puts them at particular risk of bending and falling into swimming pools, five-gallon buckets, and hampers.

Because young children have both a large head and a small body, they are at risk of becoming trapped foot first. That is, their small lower body fits into spaces—between deck railings, for example—where their head cannot fit. As a result, the lower body passes through the opening, but the child's head becomes trapped. Children have been strangled or hanged when trapped by the head in products such as playground equipment and cribs. Today, these kinds of products are designed to prevent a child's becoming trapped.

How Does Children's Development Affect Their Injury Risk?

Development—the maturity of a person's skills and biological functions, including motor skills, organ systems, and intellectual abilities—differs greatly between children and adults. The most visible developmental changes in a child are with gross motor skills. Children begin life unable to move from one place to another, but over time they gain the ability to roll, crouch, crawl, climb, walk, and run. The following three sections briefly describe children's development in terms of motor skills, biological functions, and intellectual ability and relate changes in these functions to children's risk of injury. Note that though I discuss these three functions separately, they all work together, sometimes building on one another, to increase the vulnerability of infants and young children to injury.

The Development of Motor Skills and Relationship to Injury
Motor skills can be divided between *fine motor skills,* such as grasping, holding, and turning objects, and *gross motor skills,* including rolling, crawling, and walking. Most children progress through a fairly standard series of steps as they gain both fine and gross motor skills.

cles, about nine months to crawl and stand, and nearly one year to develop the skills to take some steps.

During their second year, children master walking and then add climbing, running, and rhythmic movement, as to music, to their repertoire of skills. In their third and fourth years, children improve these skills and learn others, like ball throwing and catching.

The absence of mature muscle control and the physical inability to move out of a harmful situation are probably the major reasons for injury in the first year of life. Infants are susceptible to suffocation primarily because of their lack of muscle control and the size and weight of their head compared to the rest of their body. They can get into positions that restrict their access to air, but they cannot move out of those positions by themselves. As children gain more motor skills, they interact more with their environment, and this can lead to injuries from climbing stairs, jumping on furniture, running into sharp corners, and other activities. But their increased skill can help children get out of hazardous situations—a two-year-old will push a blanket away from his face, and a four-year-old will climb out of a toy chest.

The Development of Biological Systems and Relationship to Injury

The term *biological systems* refers to organ systems within the body; these include respiratory (breathing and lung function), cardiovascular (heart and blood vessels), digestive (eating, digesting, and eliminating functions), excretion (removing waste and byproducts of metabolism through urine and sweat), and muscle/skeleton/skin (body framework and barrier) systems. Although formed before birth, these organ systems are still immature in infants and children: infants and children have softer bones and more delicate skin than adults, infants don't have teeth, and children are unable to digest some foods as well as adults do. The immaturity of their organ systems increases infants' and children's vulnerability to many types of hazard. Injuries tend to be more serious than they would be in adults exposed to the same hazard.

Thus infants and children are more susceptible to toxins than are adults. Infants and children are likely to either absorb more or excrete less of a poison, and they are also likely to be more seriously damaged by a toxin. Lead is one toxin that causes serious injuries in children. When children ingest it, their bodies absorb a greater amount of the lead than an adult's body would, and their bones also release lead during periods of rapid growth. Since the blood-brain barrier (a layer of cells that controls the movement of substances from the blood into the brain) is immature in children, it more readily allows the transport of lead into the brain. Lead in the brain increases the risk of neurological problems, including reading and learning disabilities, decreased IQ, impaired hearing, and hyperactivity and other behavioral problems.

Infants' and children's developing muscle, skeleton, and skin systems provide less protection to internal organs than these systems do in adults. The skull plates are not fully fused at birth. The so-called soft spot on a baby's head is the location of a gap between them. The brain is more exposed in this soft area and thus is particularly vulnerable to impact injury. The bones of infants and children are also soft and subject to bending. The growth plates at the ends of bones are active—this increases the risk of permanent damage from injury. In infants and children, the outer layer of skin is thinner than in adults and therefore is a less effective barrier against cuts, scalds, bruises, and chemicals.

Teeth help us to chew foods in preparation for swallowing and digesting. Born without teeth, infants must first drink the nutrition they need and then progress to soft foods that do not require chewing. As teeth erupt, they allow children to handle different foods. A child's full set of twenty primary teeth lacks molars, which means the child can bite but cannot grind certain foods adequately. This places children at risk of choking on chunks of poorly chewed food. Childhood choking most often does involve food. Children younger than three years are at highest risk for choking, but through age five, children continue to be at risk for choking on nuts, hard candies, popcorn, raisins, hard fresh vegetables like carrots, and food with a rounded shape, like hot dogs, grapes, and gum balls. The risk of choking lessens after primary molars come in (about age three to three and a half), and it decreases substantially when the first of three sets of permanent molars begins to come in around age six to eight.

Another risk factor for choking is the fact that the eating and breathing functions share a common space at the back of the mouth. Further, in infants and young children, the opening to the airway is positioned somewhat differently from the way it is positioned in adulthood. By the time a child is about four years old, her airway has developed into the adult position. Although the overlap in eating and breathing functions continues to be a risk factor for choking in older children and adults, the anatomy of infants and young children puts them at higher choking risk. Normally, the base of the tongue closes over the opening to the airway when we swallow. The swallowed item then ends up in the esophagus, on its way to the stomach, instead of in the airway. When choking occurs, an item enters the airway instead of the esophagus. Talking or laughing (actions that require an open airway) while attempting to swallow is extremely risky because the breathing and eating systems are vying for the same space at the same time.

Infants and young children can also be at risk of injury because of their developing sense of taste. They tend to prefer sweet items, and this preference can attract them to hazards such as flavored vitamins or medicines, toys that look like candy, and sweet liquids like antifreeze. If a child puts one of these items into his mouth or aspirates it, he may be poisoned or may choke.

As infants and children grow, their organ systems develop so that their risk of sustaining the kinds of injury described here decreases.

The Development of Intellectual Abilities and Relationship to Injury

Infants and toddlers are at risk of injury because they cannot think in any organized way. Their responses are reflexive and immediate rather than the result of any deliberate thought processes. They learn from experience, which is limited initially but expands greatly as their curiosity and desire to explore become limitless. Infants and toddlers have no sense of injury risk, so their exploration is fearless. They are completely dependent, therefore, on their caregiver to keep them safe. Because language takes a long time to develop, infants cannot tell an adult how they were injured, what hurts, or what type of pain they have. Even after toddlers gain a reasonable vocabulary, they remain limited in their ability to describe events. The ability to understand and predict cause-and-effect relationships does not adequately develop until the age of five to seven years.

Intellectual immaturity puts children at risk of injury because they do not understand the injury consequences of their actions. For example, children will touch a hot stove or reach into a fireplace. They are also unable to figure out how to escape injury. A child trapped head first between the ladder rungs of a playground slide does not understand how to reorient her head and reverse her actions to free herself. A child who has been scalded by hot liquid makes no attempt to remove wet clothing; he merely screams and waits for adult intervention.

Over time, children gain the intellectual capability to assess their surroundings and their actions. With this maturity comes a better ability to anticipate what actions might lead to their getting hurt.

How Does Children's Behavior Affect Their Injury Risk?

Even before birth, babies have the ability to suck. Once born, they have a tendency to put everything in their mouth, which is the way they get their nutrition and explore their environment. But putting objects in the mouth, called *mouthing*, increases infants' and children's risk of ingestion and choking. Each object they encounter goes into the mouth, as they become familiar with its shape, texture, size, and taste. Sucking behavior typically begins to decrease when a child reaches about eighteen months of age, but mouthing continues as a means for exploration. Choking is a particular hazard for children younger than three years, and small rounded objects, like marbles and small balls, are a choking hazard for children up to age five. Balloons are a choking hazard for children as old as eight years.

When children begin to walk, at about the age of one, their access to items increases greatly, and their curiosity is heightened by all the new things within their grasp. Creativity blossoms as children imagine playmates, imitate adults, and play in new and often unforeseeable ways. Their behavior is essentially to explore, explore, explore. Because children lack a sense of appropriate behavior, they may engage in hazardous activities, such as eating plants or paint chips, licking the floor, putting erasers in their ears, and biting extension cords.

Toddlers are by nature egocentric—everything belongs to them and is about them. They can become aggressive and throw things, especially at other children. Toddlers tend to prefer solitary play, but as they develop into two-year-olds, they are more inclined to be social at play and to interact with other children. Nevertheless, at this age children are also trying to establish their independence, so they will grab toys away from other children and refuse to share. Temper tantrums are frequently a child's way to communicate what she wants. The descriptor "terrible twos" is part of our language for a reason! At this age, children are great imitators, so do not let them see you doing things that would be hazardous for them to do, like using lighters or matches.

Three-year-olds are generally sunny and agreeable individuals who are becoming more and more socialized. They begin to form friendships at this age, but the home remains the center of their world. At three years, children may express fears, such as fear of the dark or of animals.

Many four-year-olds attend a preschool, so their world now extends outside the home. They play much more physically—climbing, jumping, running—and are often outdoors. Their newfound speed and confidence increase the likelihood of injury. Among four-year-old children, the acted-out aggression often seen in toddlers and two-year-olds turns into satisfaction at observing aggression in make-believe characters, as in cartoon characters and superheroes. Therefore, a four-year-old child feels less compelled to be aggressive himself. Also, "powerful" make-believe characters sometimes help a child conquer fears, because the child feels comforted by the success of the character.

A five-year-old child is usually composed, well behaved, and very skilled. Her ability to understand the consequences of her actions is fairly well developed. Children of this age think more and do things more deliberately and systematically than do younger children.

It is no surprise that childhood injuries decline substantially after the age of five. By this age, children are far less likely to plunge fearlessly into the unknown without regard for the possibility of getting hurt. These older children are beginning to reason and to understand; an adult can explain something to them, and they remember. They can also take some responsibility for their own safety; for example, many five-year-olds can be depended upon to wear a bicycle helmet and to buckle up in the car. A child of five is beginning to come into his own. He can be better relied on to keep himself safe from harm, to listen to and remember instructions, and to think before he acts. A five-year-old can still be injured, of course, and caregivers must still watch over children of this age and older. But because children older than five years are much less likely to be injured, this book focuses on children age five and younger.

Ten Injury Prevention Strategies to Help You Keep Your Child Safe

Over years of study, injury prevention specialists have developed ten strategies to reduce or eliminate the potential for injury. Many of the strategies are aimed primarily at product designers and manufacturers. There are several good reasons for responsibility for safety to lie with the product manufacturer instead of with the product user. Manufacturers have the expertise to build safety into their product designs, and consumers have a right to reasonably safe products. Manufacturers can and should anticipate that consumers may not be able to recognize hazards, may not always understand or follow directions, may be distracted or fatigued and make bad decisions, and may improvise and introduce new hazards in the process. However, consumers must share the responsibility by using products safely. Consumers should read and follow instructions for use and warnings provided by the manufacturer. Consumers should also report injuries, near-miss incidents, and any safety concerns to manufacturers and to the Consumer Product Safety Commission.

The following ten strategies for injury prevention and control are adapted from a publication of the National Committee for Injury Prevention and Control: *Injury Prevention: Meeting the Challenge* (New York: Oxford University Press, 1989). An example is provided to demonstrate a way to implement each concept. You will find that you can easily take these actions for the benefit of your whole family, and especially for the benefit of your infant or young child.

1. Prevent the hazard.

   Example: Do not buy a hazardous product. Take note of the age grading on any toy or product purchased for a child. Age grading addresses children's ability as well as safety issues with the product. A common age label says: "Not for children under 3—contains small parts." A child younger than three years might be able to play satisfactorily with such a toy, but she would be exposed to the potential of mouthing and choking on a part small enough to lodge in the airway.

2. Reduce the amount of hazard.

   Example: When giving medicines, follow directions and measure doses correctly. Do not use household spoons as measuring devices, because they are not standard sizes. Use measuring spoons, scaled devices (which have markings to indicate the amount), and pill cutters so that the correct amount of medication is given. Scaled devices and pill cutters are available in pharmacies.

3. Prevent the release of a hazard that exists.

   Example: When setting up a playpen, portable crib, stroller, or other product that folds, read and follow the assembly instructions. Be sure to lock the product in the recommended position. Products that intentionally fold can also *un*intentionally fold, by fully or partially collapsing, if the product is not set up and locked in place correctly. Unintentional collapse can cause a child's fingers to be crushed or pinched between moving parts or a child's whole body to be trapped in an enclosed area.

4. Modify the rate or spatial distribution of the hazard.

    Example: Always restrain children in car seats and booster seats appropriate for their age and weight. If a collision or sudden stop occurs, restraints help to spread the force of deceleration over a broader area. Restraints also help prevent passengers from being thrown around inside the vehicle and possibly striking other objects.

5. Separate, in time or space, the hazard from the child.

    Example: Do not place a crib near a window. Window dressings, like blinds or draperies, often have loops in which children can become caught and subsequently hang. Also, children can fall out of windows.

6. Separate the hazard by a material barrier.

    Example: Use baby gates. Gates can prevent access to stairways, where children could fall, and prevent access to rooms like the kitchen, bathroom, or workshop, where there are hazardous materials, products, or activities.

7. Modify relevant basic qualities of the hazard.

    Example: Shorten or remove strings from toys or other playthings. Longer strings increase the risk of a child's becoming entangled and possibly being strangled.

8. Make your child more resistant to damage.

    Example: Have your child wear appropriate protection. Helmets can reduce the risk of head injury in bike incidents. Proper sunblock can help prevent sunburn.

9. Begin to counter the damage done by a hazard.

    Example: Get first aid quickly. Keep emergency phone numbers posted in view. If you think that your child has ingested poison, call a poison control center or your doctor right away, or take your child to a hospital emergency room.

10. Stabilize, repair, and rehabilitate.

    Example: Seek medical care. Get appropriate medical treatment and follow prescribed regimens for healthy healing.

As you read the following chapters, each of which discusses a daily activity, you can expect to become more knowledgeable and thorough at evaluating the safety of your children's daily environment. What you learn will help your children avoid many injuries. Some injuries will almost certainly occur, however, and thus we speak of "injury prevention *and control*." A key part of injury control is getting treatment to the injured child as soon as possible.

Here are some things you can do for effective injury control:

- Take a first aid class.
- Learn CPR.
- Learn the Heimlich maneuver.
- Have a supply of first aid items on hand.
- Post emergency phone numbers where they are easily seen.
- Call for medical help right away.

Each chapter in this book specifies measures for preventing injury and controlling injury resulting from particular kinds of hazards. By reading this book and learning about these everyday hazards and prevention measures, you will gain information to keep the children you love as safe as you possibly can.

2

🌼 Good Night, Sleep Tight

Sleep Safety

We all know that sleep is essential: it restores our energy, helps us concentrate, and keeps us healthy and feeling well. Sleep is also necessary for children's growth and development, which explains why infants and young children spend a substantial part of each day sleeping.

Although it's a good idea to check on sleeping infants and children from time to time, usually there is no reason to watch over them constantly. Creating a *safe* sleep environment for an infant or young child is an essential part of a caregiver's role, but continuously watching the sleeping child is not. For one thing, children's sleep time can be a valuable part of the day for caregivers who need rest or who are trying to tick off a list of things to do.

It's Bedtime! What Are the Safest Sleeping Arrangements?

The safest place for your child to sleep depends on her age and developmental stage. An infant is safest sleeping in a crib, because cribs are made with a baby's safety in mind. A bassinet, which is a movable basketlike bed, sometimes with legs, is another acceptable sleeping place for an infant. Bassinets are intended for infants up to about five months of age. Cribs are intended for children from birth until they are about 35 inches tall (approximately two years old) or are able to climb out. When children outgrow the crib, they graduate to a bed.

Since 1973, the U.S. government has had a mandatory safety regulation for cribs. Voluntary industry standards have also been developed more recently to address safety issues not covered by the 1973 regulation. The existence of regulations and standards is good news, because they ensure that crib designs eliminate hazards associated with past injuries and deaths. For example, to prevent an infant's being trapped, the slat spacing in cribs must be no greater than 2⅜ inches, and to prevent hanging injuries, cribs can no longer have tall end posts (finials).

The mandatory standard for cribs does not apply to bassinets, but there is a voluntary industry standard for bassinets (new in 2002). Likewise, there are voluntary industry standards for toddler beds (in effect since 1997 and revised in 2003) and bunk beds (in effect since 1992 and revised in 2001). Industry standards evolve continually; standards are made and revised as we learn more about injuries and the causes of injury. Although they may have nostalgic value, hand-me-down cribs, cradles, and bassinets can be dangerous if they belong to a different safety era. Your children should have the benefit of up-to-date safety measures. Do not use old cribs, cradles, or bassinets for children, whether at home or away from home. When in doubt about the safety of a sleep product, contact the manufacturer and ask if the product meets current standards.

Frequently, parents take newborns and young infants into their bed, because having the child in the parents' bed can facilitate feeding and encourage family bonding. However, the adult bed is not a safe place for an infant to sleep through the night, for five reasons:

1. Adult beds usually have pillows, blankets, quilts, or duvets, any of which could cover a baby's face and interfere with her breathing.
2. These beds have gaps between the mattress and the bed frame. A baby can easily be caught and trapped in one of these gaps.
3. Beds can never be pushed close enough to a wall to eliminate gaps. The greatest number of infant suffocation deaths result from babies' being wedged between a bed and a wall.
4. The adults' bed is also occupied by much larger people who can roll over, onto, or up against a baby.
5. Crib safety standards do not apply to adult beds.

Infants often fall asleep in carriers, carriages, and strollers that are made for infants but that are not specifically designed for sleep. These kinds of products are discussed in detail in the chapter about travelling with infants and children (Chapter 6). Manufacturers assume that caregivers will be nearby when carriers, carriages, strollers, and similar products are in use, so these products may not have all the safety features necessary for an infant to sleep safely while unattended. Once you get home, then, unless you can keep your sleeping baby within your view, you should transfer the baby to his crib.

Caregivers often allow infants and young children to sleep in playpens as well. Although a playpen can be a safe sleep location, I always recommend that a sleeping infant be moved to a crib. Playpens are covered by a voluntary standard, which has recently been changed to address two trapping hazards that had claimed the lives of several infants: the pocket created by drop-side mesh playpens and the V-shaped area created by collapsed playpens.

How can unsafe products be manufactured when a safety standard is in place? Say a design engineer has a new idea for a product, such as using mesh sides for a playpen. It may not be possible to fully test the safety of the new design, because the standard doesn't include provisions that are specific enough. In the case of mesh-sided playpens, the standard at the time did not contain a testing method for this new design. Unfortunately, in some cases, it is only after a product is on the market that a hazard becomes obvious. Because unsafe products can make it into the market despite safety regulations and standards, it is important for parents and other caregivers to report unsafe products, pay attention to product recalls, and use infants' and children's products that meet current standards.

On with Your PJs, Sleepyhead: Flame Resistance and Snug Fit

By federal law, infants' and children's sleepwear (sizes 0 through 6X and sizes 7 through 14) must meet flammability requirements. The flammability requirements for daywear are less stringent; this means that putting children to sleep in their daytime clothes increases the risk of burns if a fire breaks out, especially if the clothes are loose fitting. Many parents prefer cotton clothing, even though cotton is not flame resistant. These parents can put their children down to sleep in snug-fitting cotton sleepwear as an alternative to flame-resistant sleepwear. Having no loose or flowing pieces of fabric, snug-fitting clothing is less likely to catch on fire than are loose garments.

As of June 28, 2000, U.S. law requires that manufacturers attach hangtags (the tag you remove from the garment before use) and permanent labels on snug-fitting cotton and cotton-blend sleepwear to remind the consumer that these garments are not flame resistant. The hangtag says, "For child's safety, garment should fit snugly. This garment is not flame resistant. Loose-fitting garment is more likely to catch fire." The permanent label, sewn into the neck of the garment, says, "Wear snug-fitting. Not flame resistant."

A Breath of Air: Maintaining an Adequate Oxygen Supply

Normally, people breathe in and out through their nose. Air travels into the airway and down into the lungs, where blood cells take the oxygen from the air and distribute it, via the bloodstream, to all parts of the body. On the return route, blood cells carry carbon dioxide, which they exchange for oxygen in the lungs before repeating the journey through the body. The carbon dioxide returned to the lungs is exhaled.

The most serious injury associated with an infant's or young child's sleeping environment is lack of oxygen, or asphyxia. Asphyxia can occur in several different circumstances, but the cause of injury or death is always the same: insufficient oxygen. Oxygen is an essential requirement for life. The brain is very sensitive to low levels of oxygen, and when it is deprived of oxygen it can suffer permanent damage within just a few minutes. Unless access to oxygen is restored quickly, the person will die.

Sleep-related asphyxia can be divided into four broad categories:

1. Suffocation: direct covering of the nose and mouth, which prevents the intake of oxygen.
2. Hanging and strangling: pressure on the neck that compresses either or both of the airway and the blood vessels in the neck, depriving the brain of oxygen.
3. Compression and trapping: pressure, usually because the body is trapped, that interferes with the ability to breathe in and out normally.
4. Rebreathing: breathing air that has already been exhaled, which increases the carbon dioxide breathed and reduces the oxygen breathed.

Note that situations from different categories could occur simultaneously and together contribute to a child's asphyxiation. For example, an infant's chest might be compressed at the same time that his nose and mouth are covered.

A child's age affects her risk of injury from each of the four asphyxiation categories. Infants up to about six months old are at most risk of suffocation and rebreathing, because they have not yet developed the motor skills to push something away from their face or to roll away from an obstruction. Infants aged seven to twelve months are at most risk of injury from hanging, strangling, compression, and trapping hazards. These older infants have fledgling motor skills, like crouching, scooting, standing, reaching, and crawling, but they do not yet have full motor control. They can get into dangerous situations but cannot get out of them. Children aged one to three years are most at risk of hanging, strangling, compression, and trapping. One-to three-year-olds have good motor skills and are actively exploring their surroundings, but they lack the cognitive skills to recognize dangers associated with their actions. Asphyxia is the leading cause of unintentional injury death in the first year of life, but its occurrence decreases dramatically after children reach one year of age.

Because SIDS (sudden infant death syndrome) is an unexplained death, rather than an unintentional injury, it is not covered in this book. However, the recommendations provided below to reduce the risk of suffocation will also reduce the risk of SIDS.

Understanding and Avoiding Suffocation Hazards

An infant suffocates when something directly covers his nose and mouth. The infant can be lying on his back with the item on top of his face, or he can be lying on his tummy with his face in or against the item. Thin plastic bags have been and continue to be involved in suffocation deaths of infants. Any thin, nonpermeable material has the potential to cling to the nose and mouth and prevent breathing. An infant's head does not have to be inside a bag for suffocation to occur; more often a bag simply covers the face. More rarely, an infant can fall from a bed or another elevated surface and land face down on a plastic bag filled with clothes or trash.

Other fairly common articles involved in infant suffocation are pillows, fluffy bedding like quilts and comforters, soft mattresses, water beds, and fleece or down covers. Because of their softness, parents may assume these products are safe and even protective. But their appearance is deceptive. When a mother put her two-month-old daughter to sleep with her head to the side of an adult-sized pillow, she probably thought she was creating a cushioning environment. Unfortunately, she later found her daughter unresponsive, head in the pillow. The grandmother who placed a pillow in a bassinet as a mattress probably thought she was making her grandson more comfortable; she did not realize that he would sink into the soft pillow and not be able to breathe. Soft toys, like stuffed animals and soft dolls, can also cover a baby's nose and mouth, though this happens relatively rarely. As with thin plastics, infants can suffocate by being either face down on these items or face up and covered by them.

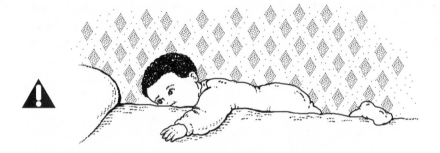

A less obvious scenario than those involving thin plastic and fluffy bedding is actually a more common cause of suffocation: an infant's being wedged between an adult bed and the wall. In fact, this scenario is the leading cause of infant suffocation death. An infant on her tummy would normally turn her head to get air, but an infant wedged face down between the bed and the wall has nowhere to turn. Infants between three and six months are at highest risk of suffocating between a bed and a wall, for several reasons:

- They tend to be taken into the parents' bed.
- They tend to scoot toward corners.
- They may be placed on the side of the bed against the wall to prevent them from falling out of the bed.
- They have not yet developed the motor skills to move away or turn over.

Infants seven to eleven months old are still at risk of harm from being wedged between a bed and a wall, but fatal incidents involving this age range are about half as common as for younger infants. For children twelve months and older, suffocation from this wedging scenario is rare.

An infant can similarly get caught between a mattress and an adult bed frame, between the cushions of a sofa or chair, between a crib mattress and the side of a broken crib, or between a crib mattress that is the wrong size and the side of the crib. The common element in these situations is a gap or space, as small as one or two inches or as

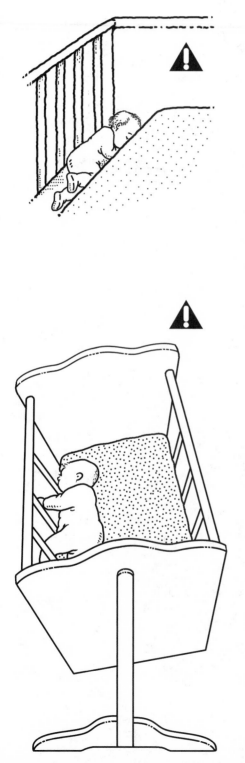

large as seven or eight inches, into which an infant's whole body or just his face moves, and he cannot get out.

Infants can also suffocate if they sleep on a surface that tilts and remains at an angle. A tilted surface forces a baby, whether face down or face to the side, into a corner or up against the end of the sleep surface. Suffocation has occurred in this way with cradles and carriers that swing or rock but fail to come to rest in a level position. In the early 1990s, the Consumer Product Safety Commission recalled a cradle that swung head to foot because of four partial or total infant suffocations that occurred when it was used. The cradle would stop rocking and remain at an angle instead of level. The baby inside would be left scrunched down in one corner, unable to move.

Suffocation can also occur when a bassinet's legs fold unexpectedly and make it collapse at one end. In such cases, a caregiver may have pushed the bassinet over a threshold or a change in floor level that forced one set of legs slightly out of position. Later, those out-of-position legs folded completely, sending one end of the bassinet to the floor. Since the bassinet standard took effect in 2002, bassinets are less likely to collapse, because those that comply with the standard cannot fold unintentionally.

The last scenario in this category is suffocation by overlying. Overlying happens when another person rolls over onto an infant. The overlying person is typically a parent but can also be a sibling. Even pets have been involved in overlying incidents. These kinds of deaths happen most often in beds, but they have also occurred in cribs and on sofas. Infants from birth to two months old are at the highest risk of suffocating from an overlying incident. For example, a mother put her young twin boys in the same crib, and one ended up pushed so closely against the other that he smothered him.

⟜ Key Actions to Prevent Suffocation

Your child will be much less likely to suffocate if you observe the following guidelines.

1. Put your baby to sleep on her back in a crib. Do not use sleep positioners.
2. Do not put pillows, comforters, or fluffy bedding in the crib. If your baby needs warmth, the best thing to do is to put her in a sleeper. If you must use a blanket, tuck it under the crib mattress and fold it well away from your baby's face.
3. Remove all stuffed animals and toys (except out-of-reach mobiles and crib gyms for babies younger than five months) from the crib while your baby is sleeping.
4. Make sure the crib mattress fits snugly—it should be the original mattress or a replacement mattress of the size recommended by the crib manufacturer. Never add a second mattress to a crib or playpen.
5. Periodically check the crib's condition and sturdiness. Make sure the side rails are firmly attached to the headboard and footboard, and make sure the mattress supports are solidly attached to the crib frame.
6. Do not take your baby into bed with you if you have been drinking or taking medication that makes you very sleepy. Avoid feeding your baby when you are very tired and are likely to fall asleep with the baby.
7. If you choose to take your baby into your bed, move the bed away from the wall, and remove pillows and soft bedding. Consider placing the mattress on the floor, away from a wall.
8. Do not put your baby to sleep on a sofa or chair.
9. Keep plastic bags (empty or full) away from your baby. Never use a plastic bag as a mattress protector.
10. Fully lock the legs of any product you use with your baby. Check the legs on wheeled products that have been pushed over a threshold or another change in floor elevation.

11. Make sure that a rocking cradle comes to rest level, not at an angle.
12. Do not put your baby to sleep with another child or a pet.

Understanding and Avoiding Hanging and Strangling Hazards

The second broad category of asphyxia involves pressure on a person's neck. This pressure can squeeze the airway closed so that

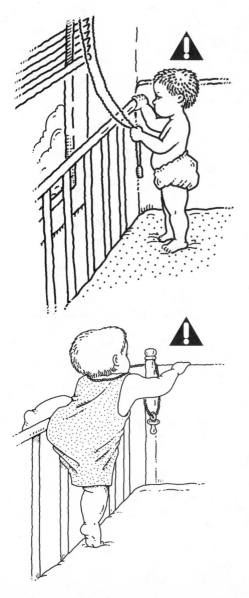

the person cannot breathe, or it can squeeze the carotid arteries so that less blood—and therefore less oxygen—flows to the person's brain. In either case, the person will quickly become unconscious. Pressure to the neck can occur either by hanging or by strangling. Although the result is the same, hanging and strangling have one key difference: in a hanging incident, the body's weight plays a role in putting pressure on the neck, whereas in a strangling incident, the body's weight is not involved.

The most common items involved in hanging incidents are blind cords, clothing, and necklaces. Any string or cord that forms a loop within reach of a child in a crib or a bed presents a hanging hazard. Two scenarios are most common: a child places a loop over her head, or an item worn around the child's neck catches on a protrusion. In each case, the child is unable to free herself. She falls, loses her balance, or simply tires and slumps so that the weight of her body puts pressure on her neck. A hanging incident can occur when a child is seated, kneeling, standing, or fully suspended and results in brain damage or death, unless the child is rescued within a few minutes.

In the past many infants were hung by a pacifier cord, worn at the neck, that caught on a crib's corner post as the child tried to climb out of the crib. This scenario happened repeatedly and spurred the mandatory requirement that pacifiers be sold without ribbons, cords, or strings attached. (A pacifier leash, a short tether that attaches with a clip, is acceptable to attach the pacifier to a child's clothing.) In addition, pacifiers must carry a warning that they should not be tied around a child's neck.

Clothing, especially with hoods or with ties at the neckline, has also caught on something sticking out from a crib and resulted in hanging. Changes in the design of crib corner posts have helped reduce the frequency of such injuries. An industry standard introduced in 1990 limits the allowable vertical space between the corner post and the side panel or the end of the crib to 0.06 inch (about 1/16 of an inch). A protrusion this small will not catch clothing or necklaces.

Children are at greatest risk of the hanging hazards described above from the ages of about seven months to three years. The younger children in this age range are at risk because they are just beginning to move about: they are learning to crouch and to pull themselves to a standing position, but they still do not have good muscle control. The older children in this age range are at risk because they are very active and are climbing in and out of their crib or bed by themselves. Across the whole range of seven months to three years, children remain unable to get themselves out of a dangerous situation.

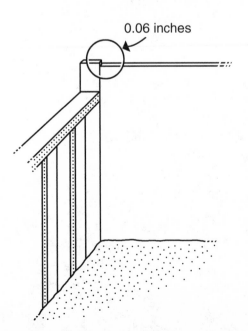

0.06 inches

One last type of hanging is called *postural strangulation* (strangling as a result of body posture). Despite its name and the fact that body position tends to be horizontal, postural strangulation is technically a hanging incident. It occurs when an infant's neck is positioned over an object or a suspended cord (as you might have on a crib gym) and the head and body weight put pressure on the neck. Infants just learning to crouch on their hands and knees (about five months old) are most vulnerable to this situation, because they can hold their position only briefly and then they slump over. If they slump over a suspended cord, they lack the muscle control nec-

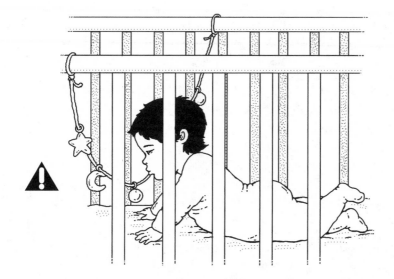

essary to lift their head. For this reason, crib gyms carry a label that says, "Remove from crib or playpen when baby begins to push up on hands and knees."

Strangling incidents, the second type in this asphyxiation category, involve items that wrap and tighten around an infant's or child's neck. Infants seven to twelve months old are at highest risk of injury from strangling incidents. The most common items that strangle infants and children, resulting in injury or death, are cords, ribbons, and strings from toys and clothing. To help minimize the risk, the toy safety standard limits string length to less than 12 inches in toys (except pull toys) for children younger than eighteen months.

Here is an example of how a strangling incident can occur. A grandmother made her infant granddaughter a lovely pink nightgown with a ribbon at the neckline, but she didn't realize that she was creating a hazard. When the mother checked on her sleeping baby, who was wearing the nightgown, she found that the ribbon had come loose and was wrapped around the baby's neck. Fortunately, it was not wound tightly, and the mother removed the ribbon completely from the nightgown.

In another example, a three-year-old boy took two remote-control toys to bed with him. Each toy had an electrical cord attached. The cords became wrapped around the boy's neck, and when he rolled over in his sleep, the cords tightened, and he was strangled.

Pressure on the neck can also happen when an infant or child is trapped in a product. This type of incident has been reported with certain playpens that collapse and create a V-shaped area that traps an infant. The infant essentially remains standing, but the playpen rails' pressure on her neck causes her to strangle. A Portland mother was called to a daycare to find her son had died in this manner. Such incidents have resulted in changes to the playpen standard. The standard now requires that playpens with central hinges and rails that move downward when folded must lock automatically when they are unfolded. This requirement prevents the formation of a V-shaped area.

⸙ Key Actions to Prevent Hanging and Strangling

There are many ways to keep your child safe from hanging and strangling situations.

1. Position the crib, bed, or playpen away from window dressings and decorative items with accessible cords.
2. Cut the cord loops on blinds and retie them as two separate cords. (Newer blinds come this way and also warn about the hanging hazard.)
3. Do not tie items, like a pacifier or jewelry, around your child's neck.
4. Do not allow your child to sleep wearing hooded clothing, a bib, or clothing with string, ribbon, or other accessories at the neck.
5. Make sure the crib has no decorative end posts that extend more than 0.06 inch (about 1/16 of an inch) above the headboard and footboard.
6. Do not hang toys in a crib by means of a cord, loop, or cargo net.

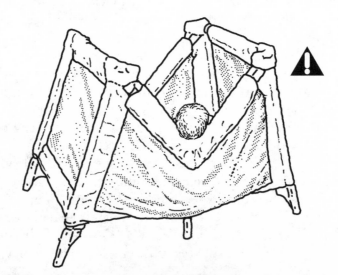

7. Remove all toys from the crib while your child sleeps, and be especially mindful of toys with a string attached. Do not allow even older children to take toys with cords to bed. Never add string to a toy.
8. Remove crib gyms and mobiles when your baby reaches five months or can crouch on hands and knees.
9. Tie bumper pad ties tightly, on the outside of the crib.
10. Make sure locking mechanisms on folding items, like bassinets and playpens, are securely locked to prevent collapse.

Understanding and Avoiding Compression and Trapping Hazards

The third broad category of asphyxia involves pressure on the chest or neck, usually as a result of a child's being trapped between a crib and adjacent furniture, or within a crib itself. Children aged twelve to twenty-four months are at highest risk of compression and trapping injuries. For example, a child may get trapped between her crib and a dresser when she climbs out of the crib. Being trapped inside a crib often involves a younger child and typically occurs when a child falls feet first into a hazardous space and his head, the largest part of the body, cannot pass through the opening. Hazardous spaces are created by any of these conditions:

- crib slats are missing, loose, or spaced more than 2⅜ inches apart
- a crib frame is damaged or loose
- mattress supports fail, causing the mattress to sag in one corner

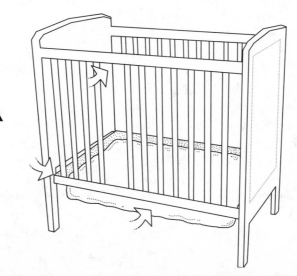

One California man thought he was being considerate and nostalgic when he offered his sister a crib that had been in his family for a number of years. The crib's slat spacing was much wider than current regulations allow, and one slat was missing. Fortunately, the baby in this case was discovered hanging outside the crib only moments after he had slipped foot first between two slats. Children aged three to twelve months are at the highest risk of becoming trapped in cribs, while older children are at risk of similar trapping incidents in toddler beds, in bunk beds, and between guard rails that do not meet current standards. There should be no more than 2.7 inches (about $2^{11}/_{16}$ inches) between horizontal sections of guard rails; 3.3 inches (about $3^5/_{16}$ inches) between a toddler bed mattress and the bed frame; and 3½ inches between a bunk bed mattress and the bed frame. To measure the space between your child's mattress and bed frame, push the mattress firmly against two sides of the frame, and measure the spaces created on the two opposite sides.

In the 1980s, mesh-sided playpens created a compression and trapping hazard when one side was left down, forming a mesh pocket. Infants rolled off, or partially off, the floor of the playpen and were trapped between the playpen floor and the loose mesh side. These playpens had been designed with a side that could be lowered to increase convenience for the caregiver. Sadly, this playpen design caused the deaths of several babies. In response, mesh-sided playpens were recalled. Today, all sides of a playpen, regardless of the material they are made of, must form a rigid right angle with the playpen floor.

Another compression and trapping hazard, termed positional asphyxia, involves a child's being trapped in a position, usually upside down, that interferes with normal inhaling and exhaling. In this scenario, an external object does not press on the chest; instead, the child's body position and the force of gravity act together to compress the chest and make it difficult for the child to breathe normally. Infants aged seven to eleven months are at the highest risk of becoming victims of positional asphyxia, although incidents are relatively rare. A positional asphyxia incident could occur if, for example, a baby falls or rolls head first into a deep cavity or container, like a hamper. In an unusual example of positional asphyxia, parents who were farm hands drove out to tend their fields and left their baby daughter sleeping in the cargo area of their SUV. When they returned, they found that the baby had moved to the side and fallen head first into the opening beside the wheel well. Though she was still alive, her breathing had been so compromised by the position that she died shortly afterward.

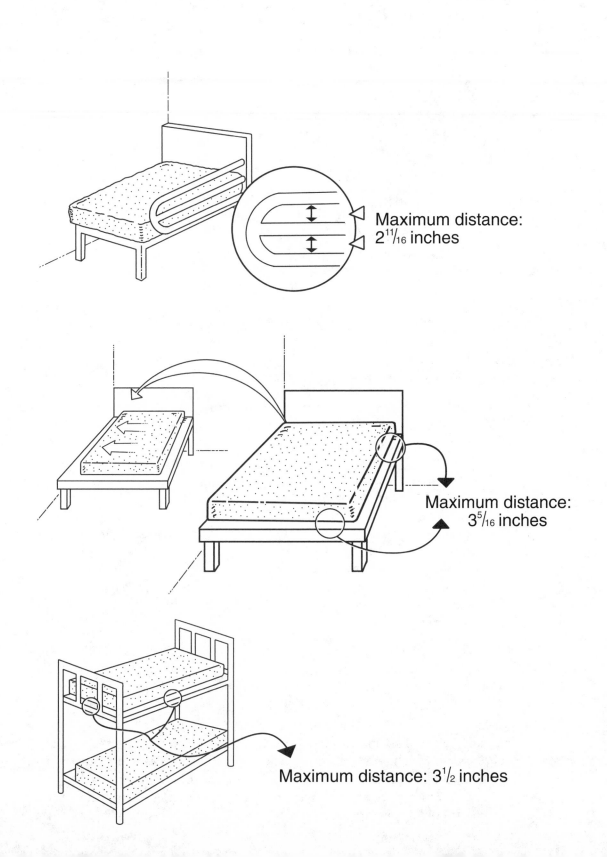

Maximum distance:
2 11/16 inches

Maximum distance:
3 5/16 inches

Maximum distance: 3 1/2 inches

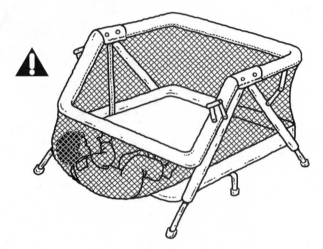

Key Actions to Prevent Compression and Trapping

Several strategies can help reduce the likelihood that your child will be hurt by compression or trapping.

1. Routinely check the condition and sturdiness of your child's crib. Look especially for damaged or shifted slats and mattress supports.
2. Routinely check the condition and sturdiness of toddler and bunk beds, especially the mattress supports.
3. Place the crib away from other furniture, like dressers and changing tables.
4. If you have bunk beds, do not allow children younger than six years old on the upper bunk.
5. If your baby is sleeping someplace other than her crib, take a careful look around to make sure there are no hampers, pails, buckets, containers, or openings into which the baby can roll or fall.

Understanding and Avoiding Rebreathing Hazards

The fourth type of asphyxiation, rebreathing, occurs when a baby breathes in carbon dioxide–laden air that he has exhaled. Infants from newborn to six months old are at the highest risk of injury from rebreathing, which typically occurs on or near soft surfaces that mold under the baby's weight. Pillows, water beds, plush quilts, soft mattresses, deep carpets, and deep fleece rugs are all examples of soft surfaces that pose a rebreathing hazard. A baby's movements, or simply her weight, can create concave areas or pockets where air gets trapped. Because the air is trapped, fresh air does not circulate into the pocket, and as the baby continues to breathe in and out, she begins to use up the oxygen and replace it with carbon dioxide. Unless access to oxygen is restored, the baby will become unconscious and will asphyxiate.

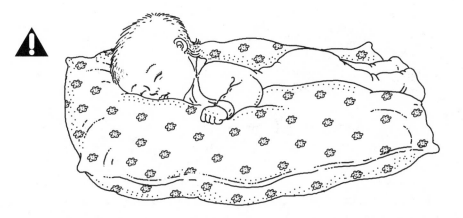

In the early 1990s, infant cushions appeared on the market and were popular with caregivers, because the cushion held a baby without additional restraints. The cushions were advertised as feeding aids, but inevitably they were used as sleep surfaces too. They were filled with polystyrene beads that moved under a baby's weight, creating indentations. Although the indentations helped prevent a baby from rolling off the cushion, they also created rebreathing spaces for a baby lying on his side or tummy. The hazard of infant cushions was so unrecognizable to the general public that even a pediatrician put his daughter to sleep on one and later found her unresponsive. The cushions were recalled and permanently banned from the marketplace because of the several deaths associated with them.

⨍ Key Actions to Prevent Rebreathing

There are several easy ways to reduce the chances that your child will be harmed by rebreathing.

1. Put your baby to sleep on her back in a crib.
2. Make sure the crib mattress is firm. Do not place your baby on a water bed, in a hammock, or on any surface into which she can sink.

3. Remove blankets, quilts, and other fluffy bedding from your baby's crib.
4. Do not use pillows around your baby—not even to keep her from rolling. Do not use sleep positioners.

Summing It Up

While infants and young children sleep, caregivers get a welcome respite from the constant vigilance required during other activities. Yet though caregivers need not constantly watch a sleeping child, they must remain alert to the sleeping environment so that the child sleeps safely. The most serious hazard associated with sleeping—asphyxiation or lack of oxygen—can be prevented if you know what items, products, and circumstances to avoid. This is true for naptime as well as nighttime sleep.

The best way to ensure a safe sleep environment for infants is to put them to sleep in a crib with no additional items (such as pillows, blankets, quilts, toys, or stuffed animals). Although bassinets and cradles are designed for infants, especially for newborns, a voluntary standard for these products did not exist until 2002. If you have a bassinet or cradle made before 2002, check that the mattress fits snugly without gaps between it and the side walls. Also check that any rocking cradle comes to rest in a level position without your having to adjust it. As your child gets older and graduates from a crib to a bed, be mindful of the potential trapping hazard posed by spaces between the mattress and the bed frame and between sections of a guard rail.

Sleep Safely Checklist

Go through the following Sleep Safely Checklist as you consider your child's sleep environment.

1. Do you lay your baby to sleep on her back?
   Babies should always be placed on their back from birth through six months, or until they can turn over by themselves. Sleeping on the back reduces the risk of suffocation as well as the risk of sudden infant death syndrome (SIDS).
2. Does your baby's crib meet current regulations?
   If you are buying a new crib, look for a label on both the

crib and the carton it comes in, specifying that the crib meets the federal regulation set by the Consumer Product Safety Commission. The retail packaging may also indicate compliance with voluntary standards: ASTM F 1169 for full-size baby cribs, ASTM F 966 for crib corner posts, ASTM F 1822 for non-full-size cribs, and ASTM F 406 for non-full-size cribs and playpens.

The crib itself must be labeled with contact information for the manufacturer. If you are reusing a crib from a previous child, call the company and find out whether the crib meets the current federal regulation and the voluntary standards mentioned above.

3. Is your baby's crib in good shape?

Routinely check the crib for signs of wear.

- Hardware should be intact and tightly fastened. If you need to replace hardware, consult the manufacturer so that you use the correct hardware. Do not use wood screws.
- Mattress supports should attach correctly in all corners so the mattress sits securely and level.
- Slats should not be loose or missing.
- The side of the crib that drops down for easy access should lock into place correctly.

4. What else is in the crib with your baby?

The baby should go to sleep with nothing else in the crib—no soft bedding, pillows, props, or toys.

5. Where is your baby's crib located in the room?

Position the crib away from windows, furniture, and decorative items.

6. Are there any thin plastic materials near your baby?

Remove all thin plastic materials (dry cleaning coverings, trash bags, grocery bags, etc.) from the area. Do not use plastic bags as mattress covers; use only covers sold for the specific purpose of covering a baby's mattress.

7. Is your baby's sleep surface level?

Avoid using sleep surfaces that could remain at a tilt and cause your baby to be pushed up against one side. This situation can happen with swinging items, like cradles, that do not automatically stop in a level position. Check that the cradle rocks or swings gently and in a small arc, and make sure that the cradle is level when it comes to rest.

8. Do you make sure not to put your baby to sleep on soft surfaces, like water beds, sofas, and hammocks?

These kinds of surfaces can mold to a baby's face or create a pocket that prevents the circulation of fresh air. Soft surfaces are also unstable; do not place your infant in an infant carrier on a soft surface, because the carrier can flip over, trapping and suffocating the baby underneath.

9. Do you know the most common pattern of infant suffocation, especially for newborn through six-month-old infants, so you can take steps to avoid this tragedy?

Babies who suffocate are found between a bed and a wall more often than in any other position. If you take your baby into your bed, position the bed well away from the wall, and move the baby to his crib when you are ready to go to sleep.

10. Does your child wear sleepwear or snug-fitting clothing to bed?

By federal law, infants' and children's sleepwear must meet certain flammability requirements. If your child sleeps in daywear, or if you prefer cotton clothing, choose snug-fitting garments.

11. Does your child's clothing have any drawstrings, loops, or loose cords, or are any of these items used as accessories?

Loops, especially around or near the neck, create a hanging hazard, because they can catch on any protrusion. Do not attach a string or cord to a pacifier, other than a pacifier leash (a short tether that attaches with a clip to your child's clothing). Do not put a child to sleep wearing a necklace of any kind.

12. If you have bunk beds, how old is the child who sleeps on the top bunk?

Do not allow any child younger than six years to sleep on the top bunk.

13. Have you checked the spacing between the mattress and frame of your child's toddler or bunk bed, and between sections of guard rails, so that you are sure they do not pose an entrapment hazard?

There should be no more than 3.3 inches (about 3⁵⁄₁₆ inches) between a toddler bed mattress and the bed frame; no more than 3½ inches between a bunk bed mattress and the bed frame; and no more than 2.7 inches (about 2¹¹⁄₁₆ inches) between horizontal sections of guard rails.

3

❦ Splish Splash

Bathing and Dressing

After the shock of being bathed in the first few months of life, many infants and children come to love bathtime. They have fun playing with water-spouting creatures, bobbing boats, waterproof books, and other bathtub toys. What child doesn't enjoy splashing and pouring water from here to there?

Despite all the hilarity of bathtime, though, there are several serious hazards. Two of these hazards are drowning and scalding, and a third, less common but no less serious, is electrocution. Once children are out of the tub and dried off, caregivers often apply lotions, ointments, or powders to them before dressing them. The skin products, the clothing, and the changing table may all present injury hazards. With care and attention, however, caregivers can minimize these hazards and prevent bathtime and dressing injuries.

Heads Up! Knowing How to Prevent Drowning

Infants and children can drown in very little water—a matter of a few inches. For very young infants who are not yet able to sit up, drowning during a bath is unlikely because the infant will probably be bathed in a small basin and held constantly by the parent or caregiver. The hazard emerges when a child graduates from a small basin to a bathtub. More than half of unintentional child drownings occur in the bathtub. From 1996 to 1999, 459 children younger than five years drowned at home (excluding swimming pools). Of these children, 64 percent drowned in a bathtub, and the others drowned in toilets, five-gallon buckets, spas and hot tubs, and other places (these will be discussed in Chapters 7 and 8).

Bath rings or bath seats have suction cups to attach to the bottom of the bathtub. These popular products are used to keep an infant upright in the tub, but they are useful for only a short period of an infant's life, in the age range of about six to nine months. Younger in-

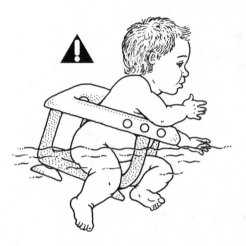

fants cannot sit up unaided, so it is too dangerous to place them in a bath ring or seat, and older children might not fit in the seat or might be able to climb out easily. Bath rings and seats play a role in helping to stabilize the slippery, wet body of an infant and also in freeing the adult's hands. However, bath rings and seats are neither safety devices nor babysitters. You cannot leave your child unattended in one of these products, not even for a moment. The suction cups can dislodge from the tub surface and cause the seat to overturn, or your baby can slip out of a leg opening or climb out of a still-engaged seat. According to data from the Consumer Product Safety Commission, children between five and eleven months are at the highest risk of drowning in association with a bath ring or seat.

A Pennsylvania mother placed her one-year-old daughter in a bath seat in the tub with the girl's two-year-old brother. The woman left the bathroom and returned to find that her daughter had somehow gotten out of the seat and was lying in the water. In Des Moines, a father found his one-year-old daughter floating after he had left her in a bath seat in the tub with her three-year-old sister. This baby girl died about a month later. In Chicago, a mother left her seven-month-old in a bath ring in a tub with about six inches of water. She left the bathroom to dress her two-year-old, and when she returned, the baby had somehow gotten out of the ring while it was still attached to the tub.

In 1999, a voluntary standard for bath rings and seats addressed certain hazards through performance requirements and labeling. As a result, bath rings and seats are less likely to tip over, the child is better secured in an upright position, and the caregiver is warned of the drowning hazard. Be aware, though, that a child cannot be left unattended in a seat simply because it meets the standard. In October 2003, the Consumer Product Safety Commission voted to establish a federal mandatory regulation for bath seats and rings, because the voluntary standard was considered insufficient to prevent drowning. As of June 2006, however, no final regulation had been published.

In some instances, children have been placed in flotation devices, such as inflatable rings and water wings, in a bathtub. One mother left her son in the bath in a flotation device and went to the kitchen to cook some rice. Thinking that her son was too quiet, she returned to check on him and found he had gotten out of the flotation device and was unresponsive in the water. Flotation devices are not life-saving devices. They are not intended for bathtub use. Even in a pool, when you use flotation devices with your child, you need to stay with him and keep him in your view at all times.

Sometimes two or more children are bathed in a tub at the same time. Parents often assume that it is safe to leave a younger child alone with an older child for a brief time. Remember, though, that children have no concept of safety or injury. A four-year-old will not know that she or her sibling can drown in water.

I cannot say it too many times: do not leave children alone in the tub, and do not let bathing children out of your constant view. In nearly all bathtub drowning incidents reported to the Consumer Product Safety Commission, there was only a brief lapse in supervision. In most cases, the parent or caregiver had reportedly left the baby in the tub for only a few minutes, to get a towel or to answer the phone. In a survey of 259 parents and guardians of children younger than five years, nearly one-third reported leaving their child alone in the bath for some period of time. Common reasons included getting towels or diapers, answering the phone, and cooking. Just over 7 percent of parents and guardians said they let their children bathe alone—in other words, get into the tub, wash, and get out of the tub without supervision—before age five.

✦ Key Actions to Prevent Drowning

You can prevent your child from becoming a victim of bathtub drowning with the following actions.

1. Do not allow a child to bathe unattended by an adult.
2. Do not leave children alone in the tub or in the care of slightly older siblings, not even for a moment.
3. While children are being bathed, do not entertain distractions—ignore the phone, the doorbell, the dog, and anything else that tries to get your attention.

4. Bring into the bathroom all the items you anticipate needing (towels, shampoo, etc.), so you do not have to leave once the bath has begun.

Hot Water: Avoiding Scalds in the Bathtub

Normal body temperature is between 98° and 99° F. Comfortable bathwater temperature should be in this range or only slightly warmer, up to 100° F. Adult skin is tougher and probably more tolerant of heat than infants' and children's skin, so a water temperature that seems comfortable to you could be too hot for a child. Use a bath thermometer to test the water temperature rather than relying on your sense of feel. You can use an instant-read thermometer or a thermosensitive card specifically intended to check bathwater temperature.

Infants and toddlers are at the highest risk of injury from bathtub scalding. Older children can also be scalded in a shower. In some cases, a parent or caregiver makes the water too hot for a child, but in many cases, a child in the tub turns on the hot water tap, or an older child enters the bathroom and turns on the hot water while a younger sibling is in the tub. Sometimes, a child climbs into a tub of hot water, and other times, an older sibling helps a child into a bath containing scalding water. Even if a child is capable of getting up and

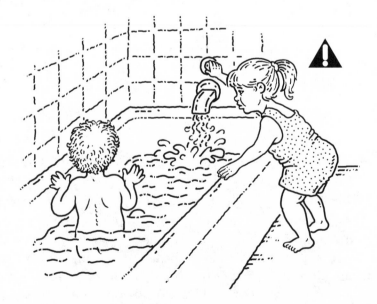

climbing out of the tub on her own, she is unlikely to do so. Children do not know enough to remove themselves from a hazard, even when they're being hurt. Instead, they cry and wait for someone to rescue them.

Bathtub scalds are among the most serious injuries, because a large part of the body can be burned, and the burn can be severe. The hotter the water temperature—and bathwater can be very hot—and the longer the exposure time, the more severe the burn will be. Note the length of time it takes for water of different temperatures to cause a full thickness (third-degree) burn:

Water temperature (° F)	Time to third-degree burn
160	instantly
140	5 to 6 seconds
125	2 minutes
120	10 minutes

These figures are for adult skin; *children's skin will burn even faster*. Serious burns require surgery to apply skin grafts and can leave children scarred physically as well as psychologically. Serious scald and burn injuries affect a whole family's emotional health.

Considerable efforts have gone into reducing the risk of tap-water scald injuries. For example, in some states, new hot water heaters are shipped from the manufacturer with lower initial settings. In a 1998 editorial in the journal *Injury Prevention*, Murray Katcher, a professor of pediatrics and family medicine at the University of Wisconsin Medical School, reported that five years after a Washington State law required hot water heaters to be preset to 120° F, and following extensive educational efforts, hospital admission rates for scalds among children declined by more than 50 percent.

Key Actions to Prevent Bathtub Scalds

You can easily keep your child, and others in your family, safe from bathtub scalds.

1. To protect your whole family, set the hot water heater lower than 125° F.
2. Consider installing scald-prevention devices, which limit the water temperature or the water flow from sink and tub faucets.
3. Rather than using your hand or elbow to measure the water

temperature of your child's bath, use an instant-read thermometer or a thermosensitive card.

4. Seat your child in the tub facing away from the faucets, so he
   is less likely to turn the hot water tap on.

5. Get organized before you begin your child's bath. Bring into
   the bathroom all the toys, towels, diapers, and other items
   that you will need, so there is no chance of leaving your child
   unattended.

Blowing the Fuse: Understanding Electrocution

Water and electricity don't mix—that message has not changed over
time, and it never will. It is wise to unplug electrical appliances in the
bathroom, and in any other room for that matter, when they are not
in use. *Even with an appliance's switch in the OFF position, electricity can flow if the unit is plugged in.*

The appliance involved most often in bathtub electrocutions used to
be hairdryers. Fortunately, hairdryer electrocutions have been reduced
dramatically since 1991, when a UL (Underwriters Laboratories)
standard took effect. This standard required UL-certified hairdryers
to have an immersion protection device to prevent electrocution if
the hairdryer was dropped into water. In the year 2000, only one
hairdryer-related electrocution was reported to the Consumer Product Safety Commission, reflecting the success of the UL standard. To
remind consumers of the electrocution hazard, hairdryers have a tag

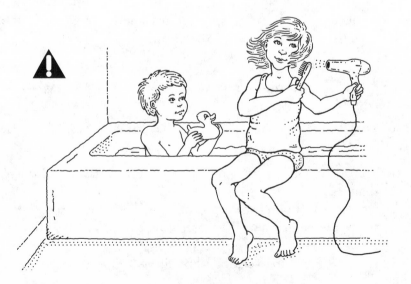

on the cord that explains how to reduce the risk of electrocution. Remember that all electric products, like radios, TVs, electric razors, and so on—even though they don't have a reminder tag as hair dryers do—pose an electrocution hazard if they fall into water or are used by a person in the tub while plugged in.

⦚ Key Actions to Prevent Electrocution

You can do several things to reduce the risk of your child's being electrocuted in the bathroom.

1. Do not allow your child to use small electrical appliances until she is at least nine years old, and even then, allow her to use appliances only under adult supervision.
2. Unplug small appliances that are not in use.
3. When you have water in the bathtub or sink, unplug all appliances or put them and their electric cords out of reach of anyone in the tub.
4. While a plugged-in appliance is in use, set it where it cannot fall or be knocked into water.

Wash Your Hands! The Importance of Good Hygiene

Before leaving the topic of bathing to discuss hazards associated with dressing a child, I would like to mention the value of good hygiene. Hand washing is one of the simplest, most effective ways to reduce the spread of illness. Teach your child to wash his hands thoroughly with soap (scrub for about twenty seconds) and rinse with warm water after using the bathroom, before helping with food preparation, and before eating. A fun way to get your child to scrub his hands for the correct length of time is to have him sing "Happy Birthday," or another jingle that takes about twenty seconds, and rinse the soap off only after he finishes singing. Remind him to wash his fingertips and under his fingernails, not just the palms of his hands.

Smooth, Soft Skin: Chemical Product Hazards

Once you've bathed your child and dried her off, you will want to get her dressed. Before putting clothing on a child, though, many parents

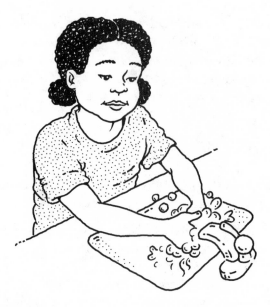

and caregivers use lotions, powders, wipes, and other products. Most products intended for external use around infants are generally safe when used as directed. These products become a hazard, however, if a child can reach them during changing and dressing. You need to keep these supplies within your reach but outside your infant's reach. The contents of many products can poison a child, while bottle caps and other small parts are choking hazards.

Baby oil, which is primarily mineral oil, poses an unusual hazard. Although baby oil is relatively nontoxic if swallowed, it can be fatal if it enters the lungs. Unintentional swallowing of baby oil can cause an infant to choke, cough, gag, or vomit, which in turn can cause some of the oil to enter into her lungs. Once in the lungs, baby oil causes pneumonitis, a potentially fatal condition. Because infants have died from baby oil–related pneumonitis, a federal law passed on October 25, 2002, requires that baby oil be sold in child-resistant packaging.

Talcum powders applied enthusiastically to a child can fill the air with particles that are easily inhaled. If you use powders, apply them gently to minimize the amount that becomes airborne and could be inhaled by your child.

⬦ Key Actions to Prevent Chemical Product Injuries

When changing or dressing your child, minimize the risks from chemical products in the following ways.

1. Keep ointments, creams, lotions, wipes, and similar products out of your child's reach.
2. Replace caps or closures on all products as soon as you are finished with them.
3. Be aware of the hazard of baby oil's entering the lungs and of the requirement for it to be sold with a child-resistant closure.
4. If you use powder for your child, apply it gently so that the air does not fill with particles.

Bumps and Bruises: Keeping a Child Safe from Falls

As infants gain mobility, they squirm, roll, kick, and twist—all of which can make changing and dressing a baby quite a challenge! Adults usually change and dress infants and young children (up to about three years old, or thirty or so pounds) on a raised surface, such as a changing table. Using a table is easier and more comfortable for the adult, but it introduces several hazards. The major hazard, of course, is the possibility of a fall. Nearly all changing-table injuries treated in emergency rooms are as a result of the child's falling from the table. Changing tables should have a raised edge to help prevent falls.

A child can get trapped in a changing table that has shelves, doors, or storage areas, but this is a relatively rare occurrence. In 2003, a combination playpen and changing table was recalled because children in the playpen could lift up the changing-table portion of the product and get their head trapped between the table and the playpen rail.

Many changing tables come with restraining straps or belts (they are required for commercial use, like in a daycare, but not for household use). There are several perspectives on the safety of using these straps. First, they may not be practical, because the restraint frequently gets in the way as you try to change and dress a child. Second, restraints have been involved in strangling incidents, when a child slips down and the restraint ends up at his neck. In these cases, a parent or caregiver has obviously stepped away, likely assuming that the strap will keep the child safely on the table.

As of July 2004, an ASTM voluntary standard came into effect for household changing tables. The key requirements of the standard are that changing tables must have a barrier and they cannot have any possible trapping areas. Changing tables can be manufactured with restraining straps, but they are not required.

⤙ Key Actions to Prevent Falls

You can easily prevent your child's falling from a changing table or other raised surface.

1. Keep one hand on your infant or toddler at all times when changing her on an elevated surface.
2. Gather all the items needed for changing and have them within your reach, so you do not have to leave your child.
3. Remember that the floor can be a good alternative for changing a baby's diaper, because there is no danger of falling.

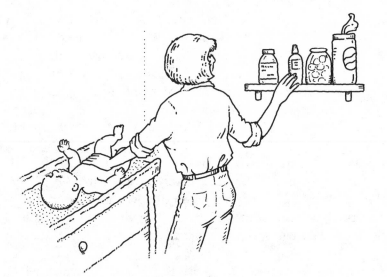

Getting Dressed: What Are the Hazards of Clothing?

Dressing a child can be a lot of fun, since the clothes are often cute, colorful, and designed with fabulous details. Dressing a child can also be awkward, though, as you try to get those arms and legs to bend the right way. As noted above, the activity of dressing poses certain hazards. But children's clothing itself can pose two serious hazards: choking and hanging or strangling.

The choking hazard of clothing comes from small decorative items, like buttons, snaps, and shoelace accessories, which can come off un-

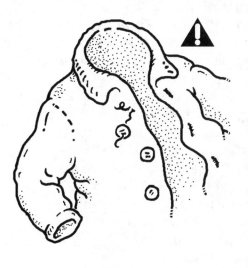

intentionally. Children's clothing and accessories are exempt from the U.S. small parts regulation, although some clothing items have been recalled because they posed an unreasonable risk of injury when a small piece, like a snap, detached. Nonetheless, be aware of the risk of small items and accessories as you buy clothes and receive gifts and hand-me-downs. Often, unsafe accessories can be easily removed. Check clothing frequently for items that are beginning to loosen, and either remove them or firmly reattach them.

The hanging and strangling hazards of clothing are associated with drawstrings, ribbons, hoods, and similar items. I'll discuss this hazard again, in a slightly different context, in the chapter about playing

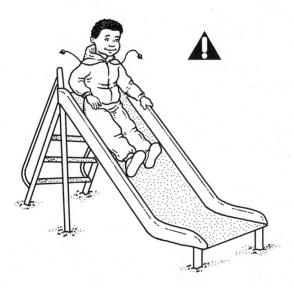

(Chapter 5). Since 1997, because of hanging incidents, an industry standard has not allowed upper outerwear, such as jackets and sweatshirts, with drawstrings at the neck to be sold for children (sizes 2T to 12). The drawstring can snag on another item, like a playground slide, or it can get caught in a moving mechanism, like an escalator. As the drawstring pulls taut, the clothing tightens at the neck, and the child quickly strangles or hangs. If you have any children's clothing between sizes 2T and 12 with drawstrings at the neck, remove the drawstrings.

As a general rule, remove all strings from the neck area of children's daywear and nightwear. Loose ties and continuous strings (that is, strings that form a loop) at the neck pose a strangling or hanging hazard. As noted earlier, fewer children hang on pacifier cords today because, by law, a pacifier cannot be sold with any kind of ribbon or cord attached. Do not tie a pacifier around a child's neck. If you want to secure a pacifier to your child, use a pacifier leash—a single short piece of material that attaches with a clip to clothing.

Drawstrings at the waist and bottom of children's upper outerwear (jackets and sweatshirts in sizes 2T to 16) are all right if they are sewn in, do not have toggles or decorative ends, and do not protrude more than three inches outside the drawstring channel when the item is expanded to its fullest width. The hazard with these drawstrings mostly applies to children aged nine years and older, so it is beyond the scope of this book, but it's worth mentioning. The reason for these requirements is that waist or bottom drawstrings on children's jackets have been caught as the children got off a school bus. With the drawstring hooked on the handrail inside the bus after the doors closed, some children were dragged alongside the bus and run over.

Loose strings and long, baggy outerwear can also be hazardous for children riding escalators. Clothing can be caught in the moving parts of an escalator and pulled taut, strangling the child or trapping a body part.

⸙ Key Actions to Prevent Clothing-Related Injuries

Keep your child safe from choking, hanging, and strangling hazards with their clothing in the following ways.

1. Check clothing for loose buttons, snaps, and other small items.
2. Either securely reattach loose items or remove them.
3. Check clothes (sizes 2T to 12), especially hand-me-downs, for strings at the neckline, and remove any that you find.
4. Before your child rides an escalator, check that she doesn't have loose cords, dangling shoelaces, or long, baggy outerwear. Hold your child's hand, and have her stand toward the center of the step.
5. Check clothes (sizes 2T to 16) for waist and bottom strings that are not sewn in, have toggles at the ends, or exceed three inches in length when the garment is fully expanded. Remove any such strings.

Summing Up

Bathing and dressing are seemingly innocuous activities, but they can result in very serious injuries and death. Perhaps part of the problem is that the hazards of bathing and dressing are not as obvious as the hazards of other activities. Parents and caregivers may not be aware that their child will be scalded in water over 125° F or that their child can drown in only a few inches of water. They also may not realize that falls from elevated surfaces can happen quickly and unexpectedly and that clothing can cause choking, hanging, and strangling injuries.

Bathe and Dress Safely Checklist

Go through the following Bathe and Dress Safely Checklist as you consider your child's bathing and dressing environment.

1. Do you stay with your child and keep him in your direct line of vision during his entire bath?

   Injury data show that children drown or get scalded when they are left unattended, even for a few minutes, in the bathtub. Ignore all distractions, including a ringing telephone, while you are bathing your child.

2. Do you use a bath seat or ring as a safety device with your child?

   Do not assume that a bath seat or ring will keep your child from drowning. You still need to stay with her and watch her for the entire time she is in the bath.

3. Is there a safe level of water in which a child cannot drown?

   The answer is no. Children have been known to drown in very little water. Even a few inches of water is not too shallow for your child to drown. Do not assume that any water depth is safe.

4. Is it all right to leave an older and a younger sibling in the tub alone, provided the older child is four or five years old?

   Again, the answer is no. Children younger than five years cannot fully understand the risk of drowning, nor will they know what to do if something happens.

5. To what temperature or temperature range is your hot water heater set?

Set the water heater to 120–125° F to minimize the risk of scalding and provide water hot enough for other household uses. If you believe you need hotter water, explore other options. Some dishwashers have a built-in heater to raise the water temperature for the wash cycle. You could also install mixing valves or limiting valves to faucets to deliver water of an appropriate temperature or flow.

6. How do you test the water temperature for your child's bath?

Use an instant-read thermometer or a thermosensitive card. If you must use your hand, place it in the water and spread your fingers. Do not use your elbow to test water temperature. The water should be around or just above body temperature, that is, 98° to 100° F.

7. To minimize the risk of electrocution injury to your child, do you unplug electrical appliances that are not in use in the bathroom?

Minimize the risk of electrocution by unplugging hairdryers, shavers, curling irons, and other appliances that are not in use. Store them out of your child's reach.

8. Do you keep one hand on your child at all times during changing or dressing on a changing table or other raised surface?

You may not want to use the changing-table restraint (or there may not be one), so keep one hand on your child to keep him from falling off the table. Even if you use the restraint, do not leave your child alone.

9. Are all your changing and dressing supplies close at hand, yet out of reach for your child?

Children will reach for and grab almost anything near them, including ointments, wipes, baby oil, medicinal creams, talcum powder, and any other items used in changing. All these products should be out of your child's reach. At the same time, they should be within your reach, so you do not have to leave your baby or take a hand off her.

10. Are you aware that baby oil can be fatal if it gets into an infant's or child's lungs?

While baby oil is relatively nontoxic if swallowed, it can be fatal if it gets into the lungs. Treat baby oil as you would any other product in a child-resistant closure. Store it out of reach of children.

11. Have you checked your child's clothing for neckline draw-strings?

Remove neckline drawstrings from all outerwear in sizes 2T to 12.

12. Have you checked your child's jackets and other upper outer-wear for waist and bottom drawstrings?

For sizes 2T to 16, make sure waist and bottom draw-strings do not have decorative ends (toggles, for example), because they can catch on or in other items. Make sure waist and bottom drawstrings are short—they should not extend more than three inches when the garment is fully expanded. In addition, drawstrings should be sewn in.

13. Have you checked your child's clothing for loose buttons, zippers, decorations, and other items?

Small items that come loose are choking hazards for young children. Check clothing, and either remove loose at-tachments or sew them securely in place.

14. Do you know the hazards for your child when he rides on an escalator, especially if he stands alone?

Make sure that your child's clothing doesn't have loose cords or long cuffs and that shoelaces are not dangling, be-cause any of these items can get caught in or between the moving parts of the escalator. Always hold your child's hand and have him stand close to the center of the escalator stair. Do not allow children to sit on escalator stairs.

4

❀ Peter, Peter, Pumpkin Eater

Food Safety

Sitting down together for a meal is a special part of the day for many families—a time to discuss plans for the day ahead or catch up on what's happened during the day. For children, mealtimes provide an opportunity to interact with other family members, learn table manners, and, of course, get the nutrition their growing bodies need.

Meals and eating come with hazards too, especially for infants and young children, but you can eliminate or minimize these hazards by supervising mealtimes and taking a few precautions.

Don't Choke: Knowing Which Foods to Avoid

Choking is a serious hazard of eating, particularly for children. The statistics tell the story: many more children die from choking on food than from choking on toys or other nonfood items. Children younger than three years, and especially those who are around one year old, are at the highest risk. Children older than four are at lower risk, but parents and caregivers must still be vigilant with this older age group.

People choke when they inhale food into their airway instead of swallowing it or when food blocks the opening of the airway. This is possible because the eating and breathing systems share some of the same space. When a person swallows normally, the tongue moves toward the back of the mouth, and the epiglottis, located at the base of the tongue, closes over the opening to the airway. This sequence allows food to enter the esophagus, the pathway that leads food to the stomach. Try swallowing and then holding it—you will notice that you can't breathe at the same time. This demonstrates how your airway is safely protected while you swallow.

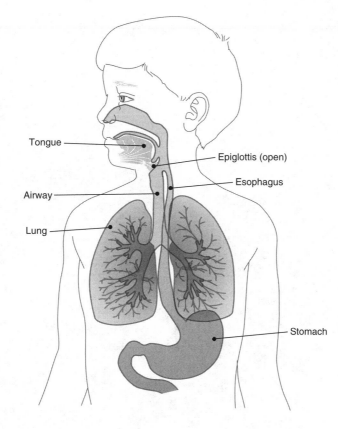

Tongue

Epiglottis (open)

Esophagus

Airway

Lung

Stomach

In spite of this protective process, people sometimes choke. How does it happen? It often happens when people laugh or talk while they eat. Laughing and talking require air, so the airway is open. Most people inhale deeply when they laugh or cry; inhaling expands the airway further, which makes the situation even more dangerous.

Children often cry, giggle, or talk while eating, so the airway is open, and possibly expanded, while food is in their mouth. One of the best ways to prevent choking is to teach your children to sit quietly while eating, to chew with their mouth closed, and not to speak until they have swallowed. Children being children, we all know that this is the ideal situation—and that ideal situations aren't the norm. Still, it is worthwhile working with your children to keep mealtimes calm and quiet. Explaining to older children why it's important to eat carefully will help them reach this goal.

When a child does choke, it means that food (or another object) has blocked the airway at one of several possible locations. Food can get

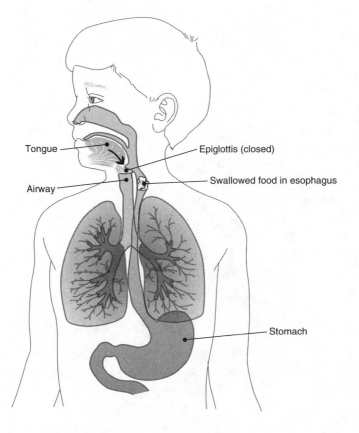

Tongue

Epiglottis (closed)

Swallowed food in esophagus

Airway

Stomach

trapped at the back of the mouth (the pharynx), the opening to the windpipe (the larynx), the windpipe itself (the trachea), a pathway leading to a lung (a bronchus), or the lungs themselves. Blockage of the airway at any of these locations can restrict a child's breathing or prevent her from breathing altogether. When a child cannot breathe at all, the blocked airway must be cleared quickly so that she doesn't suffer brain damage or death.

Choking causes a reflex cough or gag, which is frequently followed by a rapid, deep inhalation as the child tries to regain breath. A gasp such as this can draw the food (or object) farther down into the airway. Because the airway expands when a child inhales, even quite large pieces of food can enter and block the pharynx and larynx. The pharynx and larynx expand more in infants than in older children— one reason that children one year and younger are at greatest risk of choking. The airway contracts again when a child exhales.

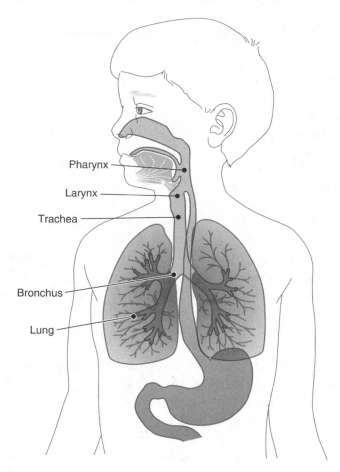

Pharynx

Larynx

Trachea

Bronchus

Lung

The size of the food determines to some extent where a child's air-way becomes blocked. Larger pieces of food, such as grapes and hot dog pieces, tend to lodge higher up in the airway, because they can't pass through the larynx. The higher up in the airway the food lodges, the more dangerous it is, because it can block the airway completely. Smaller pieces of food, such as nuts, may slip through a child's larynx and get stuck farther down in the airway. Food lodged lower in the airway may not cause a child to struggle for air in the alarming way that we think of as choking, but the situation is still serious. The food's presence can have long-term effects on the child's health, yet it can be difficult to diagnose that she has inhaled food into a lower part of the airway. Peanut halves are notorious for getting stuck in a child's bronchus or lung, where they cause irritation and sometimes an un-explained cough.

Infants are typically nourished on mother's milk, formula, and other liquids. They seldom choke on these foods, but they may gag on them. For example, a bottle with a nipple hole that is too large can deliver too much food and cause a baby to gag. Fortunately, babies generally cough and automatically correct their gagging.

Once they begin to eat solid foods, infants and children are at risk of choking as they eat. Children commonly choke because they are inexperienced at chewing and don't have all the teeth necessary to chew food well. Infants do not begin to chew until they are about eight months old. Yet by the time children are twelve months old, many of them will have been introduced to a variety of foods, some of which require more chewing skill than they possess. Children who feed themselves often try to swallow large pieces of food without taking enough time and care to chew them properly. Sometimes siblings feed each other, and the foods they offer are either inappropriate or too large to be properly chewed.

People have three types of teeth serving two different functions: incisors and canines help with biting, and molars help with grinding and chewing. Grinding and chewing prepare food so that it can be swallowed easily. Children have twenty primary teeth, which eventually fall out and are replaced by permanent teeth. Ten of the primary teeth are on the top, and ten are on the bottom; each set of ten has four incisors, two canines, and four molars.

The primary teeth come in when a child is between ages eight months and forty months (about three and a half years). A child gets his teeth in stages, beginning with the front teeth, or incisors, and later continuing with the canines and molars farther back in the mouth. This means that young children can use their incisors to successfully bite off pieces of food, but before their molars come in, they cannot adequately grind food. By age four, a child has molars, which is one reason that fewer four-year-olds choke on food than do younger children.

Children younger than five years have difficulty eating certain foods. By simply not offering these foods, you can help to prevent your child from choking. Foods that typically cause problems for young children are

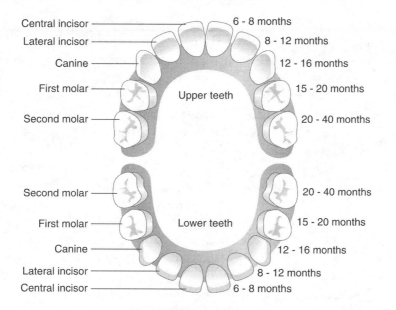

Central incisor	6 - 8 months
Lateral incisor	8 - 12 months
Canine	12 - 16 months
First molar	15 - 20 months
Second molar	20 - 40 months

Upper teeth

Second molar	20 - 40 months
First molar	15 - 20 months
Canine	12 - 16 months
Lateral incisor	8 - 12 months
Central incisor	6 - 8 months

Lower teeth

- foods with rounded shapes, like grapes and hot dogs
- hard items, like hard candy, nuts, and raw hard vegetables
- popcorn
- raisins
- fruits with a pit
- gobs of peanut butter

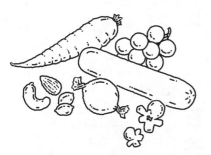

Round or cylindrical foods can plug the airway like a stopper in a bottle, and thick foods, such as peanut butter, can mold to the airway. Hard candy and fruit pits can be slippery and difficult to control in the mouth.

When children are fed or try to eat inappropriate foods, the result can be devastating. A ten-month-old boy died when his two-year-old brother fed him a hot dog. The hot dog completely blocked his upper airway. A three-year-old died while eating a peanut butter sandwich. A puttylike mass of bread and peanut butter plugged her upper airway. A ten-month-old was in bed with her mother, who was eating Spanish limes, a small fruit with a grapelike texture and a large pit. The baby put a pit in her mouth, and it completely blocked the trachea. When she stopped breathing, her mother called for help.

For many years, studies of childhood food choking have consistently found these foods listed above to be the cause of choking. One study from 1979 to 1981 examined choking cases in forty-one states, which included 87 percent of U.S. children aged newborn to nine years. This study found that four foods—hot dogs, candy, nuts, and grapes—together contributed to over 40 percent of all food deaths in which the type of food was identified. In a little over half of the cases, the foods involved were round or cylindrical. For one-year-old children, a wide range of foods caused choking, including meat products and carrots. For children up to the age of two years, apples, biscuits, and cookies caused choking deaths, and at age two years, peanuts and grapes were also a problem. At age three, the total number of deaths dropped, but the number from choking on hot dogs increased.

Another food to be wary of is an Asian import food known as a mini-gel snack. In recent years, mini-gel snacks have been associated with choking deaths, even among older children and adults. The product involved was a single-serving gel, packaged with some liquid in a container similar to those used for single servings of liquid coffee creamer. A mini-gel snack was eaten by peeling back the foil lid and sucking out the whole gel in one slurp. The product was rounded or conical and was made with konjac, a thickener that made the gel very tough, difficult to break apart, and slippery. Konjac-containing gels have been banned in the United States by the Food and Drug Administration (FDA) since October 2001. They have also been banned in many other countries.

If you purchase a mini-gel snack, check the ingredient label to be sure it does not contain konjac (also called konnyaku, yam flour, or glucomannan). In addition to being made without konjac, newer versions of the product usually have irregular and larger shapes. These new shapes are better because they make it unlikely that the whole piece of gel will be taken into the mouth at once. Still, these gel snacks typically have pieces of fruit embedded in them, so they are not suitable for children younger than three years.

The results of studies such as the one mentioned above are both alarming and sad. Fortunately, you can help to keep your child safe from choking by offering her only appropriate foods, cut into suitable sizes and shapes. Explain to older children that their younger siblings and friends can't yet chew well enough to eat some of the foods they are eating. Also, be sure to keep an eye on toddlers who may try to feed an infant.

Finally, as every parent knows, children routinely put nonfood objects in their mouth. In fact, this is often the first thing young children do when they find a new object, whether large or small. If a child chokes on a nonfood object, it can block the airway at any of the locations mentioned earlier. If a child swallows a nonfood object, it typically passes from the body in a bowel movement. But sometimes a swallowed object can lodge in a child's esophagus and press on the trachea. This seems to happen most often with objects such as large coins, belt buckles, and safety pins. Although this is not actually choking, it is still serious. Injuries from swallowing nonfood objects can be difficult to diagnose because the child may complain only intermittently of pain or discomfort.

Key Actions to Prevent Choking

You can do several things to reduce the risk that your child will choke while eating.

1. Feed your child only foods that she is able to chew and swallow. This often means preparing the food correctly for her age.

   - Birth to six months: breast-fed or bottle-fed breast milk or formula; if you use a bottle, choose nipples with a hole that is not too large, and discard nipples that are brittle or cracked.
   - Four to six months: baby cereal
   - Six to seven months: pureed fruits and vegetables
   - Seven to eight months: chopped or mashed finger foods, like cooked vegetables cut into strips; O-shaped oat cereal
   - Eight to ten months: ground meats, macaroni, and crackers
   - Ten to twelve months: table food cut into small pieces, but not rounded shapes; soft cheeses, yogurt, and ripe bananas
   - One to five years: smooth peanut butter spread thinly, never in a glob
   - Never offer nuts, hard candies, popcorn, food with rounded shapes, raw carrots, celery, or other hard vegetables to children younger than five

2. Teach your child to sit—not walk or run—while eating.

3. Teach your child to chew and swallow with her mouth closed.
4. Teach your child not to speak until after she has swallowed her food.

First Aid to Help a Choking Child

You know which foods not to give your child, and you know how to prepare foods so they aren't a choking hazard. Yet even with all the knowledge, planning, and watchfulness in the world, it is still possible that your child might choke on her food. Fortunately, many choking episodes resolve themselves; for example, if the child coughs and clears the airway, the choking incident ends safely. If a choking episode doesn't resolve itself and your child can't breathe, can't make any sounds, or becomes unconscious, you can be a great help if you know what to do and if you act quickly. The following four actions could help you save your child's life.

1. Know that what you do differs with your child's age.
2. Learn and practice CPR (cardiopulmonary resuscitation).
3. Check with your doctor, the local Red Cross, or the American Academy of Pediatrics for the latest first aid methods.
4. Keep first aid information where you can readily access it; for example, paste it or tape it securely to the inside of a kitchen cabinet door.

The American Academy of Pediatrics (AAP) and the Heimlich Institute both provide recommendations for helping a choking child. There are some differences between their respective recommendations for children younger than one year. The recommendations of both associations are summarized below so that you know what they are.

For a child younger than one year who is choking and unable to breathe, cough, cry, or speak, the AAP recommends using a combination of back slaps and chest thrusts.

- Hold the child face down and head down, and give five back slaps.
- Then lay the child face up and give five chest thrusts.
- Alternate these two actions.
- Call 911 if you are not successful in clearing the airway after one minute.
- If the infant becomes unconscious, begin CPR.

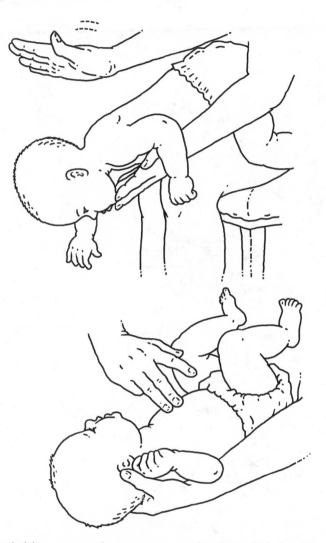

For a child younger than one year, the Heimlich Institute recommends that you use a modified Heimlich maneuver and does not recommend back slaps.

- Lay the child on a firm surface, and kneel or stand at the child's feet, or hold the child sitting on your lap facing away from you.
- Place the middle and index fingers of both your hands below the rib cage and above the navel.
- Press into the child's upper abdomen with a quick upward thrust. Be very gentle, and do not squeeze the rib cage.

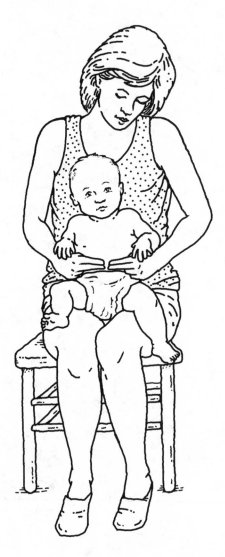

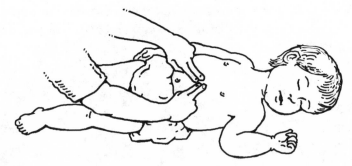

- Repeat this action until the object is expelled.
- If the child has not recovered within one minute, call 911, and proceed with CPR.

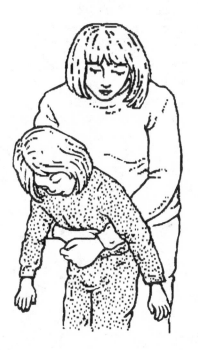

For a child older than one year, the AAP and the Heimlich Institute make essentially the same recommendations.

- From behind, wrap your arms around the standing child's waist.
- Make a fist and place the thumb side of your fist below the ribcage and just above the navel.
- Grasp your fist with your other hand and press into the upper abdomen with a quick upward thrust. Do not squeeze the ribcage. Confine the force of the thrust to your hands.
- Repeat this action until the object is expelled.
- If the child has not recovered within one minute, call 911, and proceed with CPR.

The Heimlich maneuver is named after Dr. Henry J. Heimlich, who, in 1974, described the maneuver as forceful upward thrusts with the fist, directed toward the diaphragm. The idea is that this action forces air out of the lungs to dislodge the object blocking the airway. You need to be gentle when performing the Heimlich maneuver on a child, because injuries can result, including broken ribs and ruptured internal organs.

Sternal thrusts (quick pushes in succession on the breastbone) are usually used in CPR. They apply pressure to the trachea to dislodge the object blocking the airway.

Doing a finger sweep in the mouth is useful if you can see the object. Trying to pull an object out, though, may actually force it farther down the airway.

That's Hot! Avoiding Burns and Scalds

Burns and scalds are another serious hazard during meals and anytime you heat foods or liquids. The hot food or liquid as well as the hot container on the tabletop or countertop can harm young children. But you can easily avoid burns and scalds by taking some simple precautions when handling hot items around children—see below.

A contact burn, also called a thermal burn, typically occurs when a child touches a hot surface. Contact burns most often affect fingers and hands. Scalds typically happen when hot foods or liquids are spilled or knocked over. Scalds tend to affect a larger part of the body; for example, when food or drink is spilled at the table, a seated child's lap and legs may be scalded. Because scalds often affect a large area of a child's body, they tend to be more serious injuries and require hospitalization more often than contact burns do. Hot foods and liquids can also scald a child's mouth and esophagus as she eats or drinks. (Burns and scalds from cooking, rather than from eating, are dealt with in Chapter 8's section on kitchen hazards.)

Young children, especially those younger than two years, are at the highest risk of burns and scalds for two reasons. First, they do not understand "hot" and the consequences of touching or spilling hot items. Young children will reach for and grasp at anything. Second, they do not have well-developed manual skills. Young children drop things, spill things, and knock things over all the time.

Children are particularly vulnerable to serious burns and scalds because of their small size: a spill will cover a larger part of their body than it would of an adult's body. Children also have thin, delicate skin, so more layers of skin can be burned more quickly.

Key Actions to Prevent Burns and Scalds

Fortunately, there are several easy actions you can take to reduce the chances of your child's being burned or scalded by hot foods and liquids.

1. Do not overheat food.
2. Shake or stir well all heated foods and liquids to get rid of hot spots. (Note that microwave cooking often creates hot spots in food. Make sure to stir food, to distribute the heat.)
3. Place hot dishes and containers out of your child's reach. If he eats in a high chair, place the hot dish or container on the table. If he eats at the table, place the hot dish or container more than two feet away from him—seated two-year-olds can reach to nearly 27 inches, which is a little over two feet.

4. Do not use placemats or tablecloths, because your child can easily pull on them and overturn food or drink.

If your child does get burned, cool the burned area under cool running water for ten minutes or longer, or use wet sterile dressings. Do not put ice, butter, or any other kind of oil on the burn. Check with your doctor.

If your child gets scalded, cool the area or cool the wet clothing by soaking it with water. Remove clothing that is not stuck to the skin. If the clothing is stuck, then leave it on your child, because the skin will come off with the clothing. Her clothes will need to be removed by a health care professional. Check with your doctor, or call 911.

Safe Seating: What Are the Hazards of Carriers and High Chairs?

The seat your child occupies while he eats is another safety issue for you to think about. Again, once you know the hazards and how to avoid them, you can help to keep your child safe.

Children inevitably squirm and shift while they eat (or while they resist eating!). Their movements may lead them to slip or fall from their seat. Infants' and children's seating has three hazards: an infant and her carrier together can fall off the surface where they were placed, a child can get trapped between a high chair's seat and tray, and a child can fall out of a high chair or off a seat. Hand-held infant carriers, high chairs, and hook-on chairs all have standard safety features that address these hazards, but the products must be used correctly for the safety features to be effective. The most common safety problem is failing to fasten the restraint or seat belt provided with the carrier or chair.

You are most likely to feed an infant while holding him in your arms or in a carrier. Carriers are often placed on an elevated surface, like a table, for convenience, but a baby's movements can cause the carrier to slide toward the edge and fall off. A fall from an elevated surface is the most common injury pattern for infants in carriers, and the result can be skull fractures and other serious injuries.

A child becomes trapped between a high chair's seat and tray when he slips downward through the leg opening and his neck is stopped by the chair's tray. Sometimes referred to as "submarining," this type

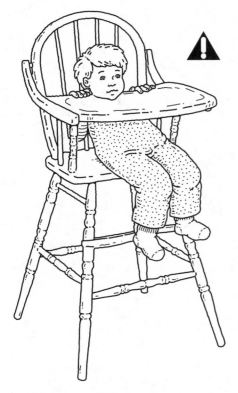

of trapping may strangle a child as his neck is pushed up against the tray or restraint. A trapped child must be rescued quickly to avoid brain damage or death.

As a child gets older, she may try to stand up in her high chair. Some chairs hook onto the table, and as a child grows and gets stronger, she may dislodge the chair from the table by pushing against a table leg with her feet. When a child begins to sit in a regular seat, she may try to stand on the chair or may tip it over. Falls in any of these cases could cause serious injury, so be sure to use the chair's safety features correctly and explain to older children the importance of sitting still while eating.

Key Actions to Prevent Trapping and Falling

You can keep your child from becoming trapped or from falling during mealtimes with the following actions.

1. If you place a hand-held carrier on an elevated surface, place it well away from the edges, and keep one hand on the carrier. It is safer to set the carrier on the floor.
2. Secure your child in a high chair using the seat's restraint system. The restraint helps to keep him seated in the correct position.
3. Push the tray table of a high chair close to your child, and make sure that it locks in place.
4. Attach hook-on chairs away from table legs and other surfaces that your child could use her feet to push off from. Do not put a regular chair under the hook-on chair.
5. Stay with your child so you always have him in view, no matter which seating system you use.

A Spoonful of Sugar: Getting the Medicine Down Safely

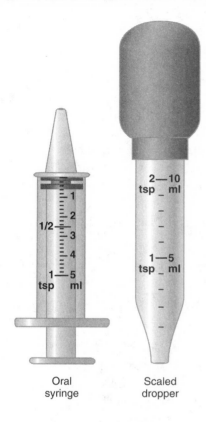

2—10
tsp _ ml

1—5
tsp _ ml

1/2

1
2
3
4
1—5
tsp   ml

Oral
syringe

Scaled
dropper

Taking medication is not really eating, but I cover it in this section because medications often need to be taken with food, and the topic is extremely important. Nobody likes being ill and nobody wants to take medicine, least of all a child. Unfortunately, though, getting sick is a nearly universal experience, so we all need medicine from time to time. When a doctor has prescribed medication, it is very important to take the correct amount at the correct intervals and for the complete period of the prescription.

Overdosing on a medication can result in poisoning, and underdosing can lead to ineffective treatment of the illness. Always give each dose of medicine to your child using something that measures the dosage accurately. For example, use a scaled oral syringe (oral syringes do not have a needle) or a scaled dropper ("scaled" means that it has markings to allow you to measure to a "fill" line). Do not measure medicines using ordinary tableware—teaspoons and soup spoons in a tableware set are not standard sizes.

✦ Key Actions to Prevent Overdosing or Underdosing Medicines

You can reduce the likelihood of overdosing or underdosing your child's medication in the following ways:

1. For medications that do not come premeasured or that are not packaged with something to measure them accurately, buy a scaled measuring device at your pharmacy. Ask the pharmacist to assist you in buying the correct item.
2. Always give your child the entire prescription of medication, even if she feels better before the medication is finished. The only exception is when your doctor or pharmacist tells you otherwise.

3. If you believe that your child has taken too much medicine, call the U.S. National Poison Hotline (1-800-222-1222) for guidance.

Summing Up

Eating together at mealtimes is a highlight of the day for many families. When you have young children, mealtimes can also be hectic and demanding. Children require special attention to stay safe while eating, but by remaining watchful and following certain precautions with food, hot items, and seating arrangements, you can ensure that mealtimes are as safe as possible.

You can greatly reduce the chance of your child's being injured while eating if you

- monitor the types of foods given to your child so they are appropriate to his ability to chew and swallow
- keep your child seated during meals
- stay with your child during the feeding

Use safety straps or restraint systems to help keep younger children seated and to reduce the risk of their becoming trapped or falling. Correctly attach hook-on chairs to help lessen the risk of falls. Also, be aware that infant carriers can easily slip from elevated surfaces.

Eat Safely Checklist

Go through the following Eat Safely Checklist as you consider your child's eating environment.

1. Do you check the nipples of baby bottles for wear and brittleness?

    Nipples do wear out. They can become brittle or cracked over time. Examine nipples, and discard any that show signs of wear. Your child can choke on pieces that break off a worn nipple.

2. Do you know why children younger than age five tend to choke on foods?

    Young children choke primarily because they do not have the teeth necessary to chew and fully prepare food for swallowing. When they get front teeth, they can bite off large pieces of food, but until they get molars, they cannot grind and chew the food properly.

3. Are you aware of the shapes and foods most commonly associated with choking in children younger than five years?

   The most common and most dangerous shape involved in choking incidents is round. The foods most likely to cause a child to choke are hot dogs, nuts, grapes, and hard candy. Hot dogs, grapes, and hard candy tend to be slippery and difficult to control in the mouth. They can start moving toward the back of the mouth before a child is ready to swallow.

4. Do you know why rounded shapes, such as hot dogs, grapes, and hard candy, are so dangerous for children?

   Rounded shapes form effective plugs in the airway and are difficult to dislodge.

5. Can you ever give a hot dog, sausage, grape, or similar item to a child younger than five years old?

   Ideally, you will have other foods available. But if you must offer these foods, give them only to a child older than three years. Always remove the casing from hot dogs and sausages and the skin from grapes, and then cut the food into tiny cubes, not round shapes.

6. Does your child sit at the table to eat rather than walk around while eating?

   It is safer for your child to be properly seated for meals. This way, you can watch her better, monitor the mouthfuls she takes, and teach her to chew and swallow before talking.

7. If your child is in a high chair, booster chair, or hook-on chair, do you use the seat restraint?

   Securing your child in a seat reduces the risk that he will climb or fall out of his chair or that he will slip beneath the tray or table and become trapped.

8. Are the foods and liquids you offer your child heated evenly to a warm—but not hot—temperature?

   Your child can be scalded by eating or spilling foods that are too hot or that have hot spots. Microwaves can heat foods unevenly, so stir or shake foods to ensure even warmth before offering them to your child. Keep dishes of hot foods out of your child's reach during feeding.

5

🌸 It's Playtime!

Toys, Games, and Playgrounds

A child's work is to play and have fun and, along the way, to learn a few things. In fact, playing includes all kinds of activities that help a child hone motor, cognitive, and social skills. The real goal for children, though, is to play with toys and games and at playgrounds for pure enjoyment, whether they play alone or with friends.

The type of play that children engage in varies greatly with their age. For young infants, play is mostly about seeing objects and hearing sounds. Many infants are mesmerized by things like crib gyms, crib toys, mobiles, and music or sound makers. As infants gain manual ability, they love to grasp objects around them and, of course, put these objects in their mouth. Rattles, stuffed and sewn items, and stacking toys provide hours of entertainment. As soon as children begin to stand and walk, push and pull toys become popular, and as they gain more physical skills, children love nothing more than playing with ride-on toys, wind-up toys, and balls.

At around two years, children grow into fantasy play, and they begin to act out whole scenes with action figures, dolls, and other toys. Fantasy play persists for many years. Children's creative side also emerges at about two years, as they play with crayons, finger paints, and other art supplies. By about four years, children have fairly well developed fine motor skills, enabling them to enjoy games with little pieces. Mobile children of all ages love to play outdoors as well, no matter whether they're at a playground, a beach, a park, or in the backyard. Their desire to explore leads children to play with anything and everything, plaything or not. They play with things in myriad ways, regardless of how the toy or item was intended to be used.

Because play is such a broad area, I can't cover every type of injury hazard in these pages. So I discuss the most common hazards associ-

ated with playing, as well as those that are less common but have potential to cause severe injury or even death, and I tell you how you
can prevent or minimize the risk of your child's being harmed while
he plays.

Teddy Bears, Fire Engines, and Soccer Balls: Choosing Safe Toys

An immense variety of toys crowds store shelves today. How do you
decide which ones are safe for your child to play with? Fortunately,
most toys are safe, thanks to U.S. government regulations and industry standards. The Consumer Product Safety Commission regulates
rattles, small parts in toys intended for children younger than three
years, lead content of paint and surface coatings on toys, electrical
toys, labeling for art supplies, and bicycles. It is mandatory for toy
manufacturers to comply with these regulations. The Commission has
the authority to recall products that fail to conform to its regulations.
If it determines that a product poses a substantial risk of injury, even
if there is no applicable regulation or standard, the Commission can
recall that product as well. The Commission can also impose penalties on manufacturers or distributors for their failure to abide by the
regulations.

A voluntary industry toy safety standard has been in place since
1986, and since then it has undergone several changes and expansion
in coverage. The standard addresses a broad variety of hazards for
many different types of toy. Most toys, especially those made or imported by reputable U.S. companies, are tested against this industry
standard before they are marketed, but compliance is not mandatory.

Though most toys are reasonably safe, there will always be some
that are hazardous by design, that do not meet standards, or that are
not safe despite meeting standards. Sometimes a product has hazards
that don't appear during safety testing, because there is no testing pro-
cedure to identify those particular hazards. Other times, a hazard becomes evident because of the unanticipated way a child plays with the
toy. Consumers should report unsafe products to the Consumer Product Safety Commission. You can file a report on the Commission's
website (www.cpsc.gov), or you can call its hotline at 1-800-638-
CPSC (1-800-638-2772).

The industry toy safety standard recommends that manufacturers provide age grades on toys. Age grading generally establishes a lower age limit, the minimum age a child should be to use the toy as intended. Sometimes, age grading also includes an upper limit, thus establishing the most appropriate age group to use the toy.

The standard also requires that certain toys have safety labeling. Safety labeling explains a hazard that exists if the toy is used by a child outside the recommended age group. A common safety label reads, "Warning—Choking Hazard—not for children under three." As you choose toys and playthings for your children, read the age and safety labeling to find out (1) the appropriate user age from an expected skill level, and (2) the hazards associated with giving the item to a child outside the recommended age.

True, children vary in their skills, and you may anticipate your child's development and want to buy toys for her to grow into. Nonetheless, keep in mind that there are different safety requirements for toys intended for different age groups. These requirements are based on the expected capabilities and limitations of children according to their age.

The following list tells you the types of toys that require age labeling or safety labeling and explains why the labels are needed.

1. Crib gyms, crib exercisers, and activity toys intended to be strung across a crib or playpen by means of string, cord, elastic, or straps must be age graded for infants up to five months and must be labeled "WARNING: Possible entanglement or strangulation injury. Remove toy when baby begins to push up on hands and knees." This labeling requirement came about because injury data showed that when infants are beginning to lift themselves to a crouching or crawling position, they don't yet have sufficient strength to control their movements and can fall onto or flop over a crib gym or toys suspended across their crib (see illustration on p. 33). Since a baby cannot lift his head off the cord or suspended material, the weight of his head puts pressure on the front of his neck, and he is strangled.

2. Mobiles must be age graded for birth to five months and must be labeled "WARNING: Possible entanglement injury. Keep out of baby's reach." Mobiles intended to be attached to a crib or playpen must also be labeled "Remove mobile from crib or playpen when baby begins to push up on hands and knees." These requirements are intended to prevent infants'

getting tangled in the strings or cords that suspend items from mobiles or that are part of the mobile itself. Fingers are at the highest risk of being wrapped tightly, cutting off blood supply. More severe injuries include strangling or hanging when a child's clothing gets caught on a protrusion from the mobile, such as a clamp or screw.

3. Toys intended to be strung across strollers or carriages by means of string, cord, elastic, or straps must be labeled "WARNING: Possible entanglement or strangulation injury when attached to a crib or playpen. Do not attach to crib or playpen." This label reminds parents and caregivers that suspended toys that are safe for a seated child may pose a tangling or strangling hazard for a child lying or crouching in a crib or playpen. Stroller and carriage toys should be used only with strollers and carriages.

4. Toys intended for children at least three years old but younger than six years and containing small parts must be labeled "WARNING: CHOKING HAZARD—Small parts. Not for children under 3 yrs." The labeling requirement for toys with small parts began when injury data showed that young children were playing with older children's toys and choking on small pieces that were legitimate parts of those toys. Toys intended for children at least three years old but younger than eight years and containing small balls or marbles must be labeled "WARNING: CHOKING HAZARD—Toy is [or contains] a small ball [or marble]. Not for children under 3 yrs." A small ball is defined as having a diameter less than 1¾ inches. The small ball and marble labeling requirements are in place because these products pose a serious choking hazard. They can easily block the back of the throat or the opening of the airway and are extremely difficult to dislodge. Marbles can be a choking hazard even for children as old as five years. Compared with other shapes, toys with round shapes pose the highest risk of choking death.

5. Latex balloons and toys and games that contain a latex balloon must be labeled "WARNING: CHOKING HAZARD—Children under 8 yrs. can choke or suffocate on uninflated or broken balloons. Adult supervision required. Keep uninflated balloons from children. Discard broken balloons at once." The Consumer Product Safety Commission reports that between the late 1980s and today, latex balloons have caused

more choking deaths of children younger than five years than any other product. Children through age eight are at risk of choking on balloons, but children younger than one year are especially at risk. Inflated balloons are not the problem; it's uninflated and broken balloons that cause the choking hazard. If a child inhales in preparation to blow up a balloon or puts a piece of broken balloon into her mouth, she can draw the balloon or piece of balloon to the back of her throat, where it "molds" in place. Balloon pieces are extremely difficult to extract.

6. Simulated protective devices, such as toy helmets, must be labeled to inform parents and caregivers that these devices are toys and are not intended for injury protection. This requirement alerts adults not to expect their child to get true injury protection from such a device. The only products that provide injury protection are those that meet specific requirements or standards, such as the bicycle helmet standard.

7. Flotation toys, such as inflatable rings and water noodles, must be labeled "WARNING: This is not a lifesaving device. Do not leave child unattended while in use." This labeling requirement is to prevent adults from mistaking toy flotation devices for true lifesavers or life jackets. The only actual lifesaving devices are those approved by the U.S. Coast Guard.

8. Toys with sharp points or edges that are functional—for example, a play sewing machine with needles—must be labeled to warn of their sharp contents. Toys with functional sharp points and edges are intended for children at least four years old. The label informs parents and caregivers of the potential hazard and enables them to decide whether they want to purchase the toy and whether the toy is appropriate for the particular child and household.

9. Art materials, such as crayons, paints, glues, and craft supplies, must be tested for chronic toxicity (that is, the ability to cause cancer, nerve damage, or birth defects) and labeled to state their compliance with applicable standards. The Labeling of Hazardous Art Materials Act, passed in 1988, established this requirement. Some art materials contain hazardous chemicals that could have toxic effects when used over long periods of time. Since 1990, such art materials must be labeled to indicate the possible long-term effects. Children's products are not allowed to contain any hazardous

chemicals. Look for the label stating, "Conforms to ASTM D-4236" to be sure a product has been tested and found to be not toxic.

To help parents find appropriate toys for children with special needs, the Toy Industry Foundation has worked with the American Foundation for the Blind and the Alliance for Technology Access to publish a guide called *Let's Play: A Guide to Toys for Children with Special Needs.* The guide matches toys with children who may find them most enjoyable. It includes toys for children with physical impairment, hearing impairment, blindness or low vision, and developmental disabilities, including Down syndrome and autism. The 2006 edition of the *Let's Play* guide is available from the Toy Industry Foundation at www.toy-tia.org, or you can e-mail tifinfo@toy-tia.org and request a copy.

Put Away Your Toys: Safe Toy Storage

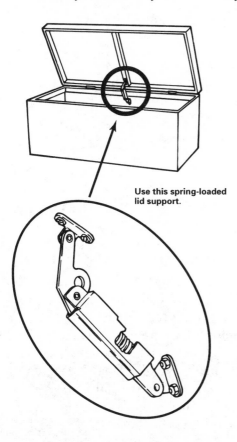

Use this spring-loaded lid support.

Choosing appropriate toys for your child is a first step; the second is storing them safely in your home. Parents and caregivers commonly use toy chests and storage shelves, both of which have some hazards that can be easily avoided. With toy chests, the lid can fall closed on a child who is leaning into the chest. If the child, trapped between the lid and the toy chest, is unable to free himself, he can strangle. A child may also climb into a toy chest (or another closed space) and be trapped inside. Without adequate ventilation, the child will suffocate. An industry safety standard addresses both of these hazards with toy chests. The standard requires toy chest lids to have a hinge or other mechanism that prevents them from falling closed. The standard also requires that toy chests have ventilation holes of a certain size and location.

If you use other storage boxes or bins in lieu of a toy chest, be aware that they might present the lid-trapping and suffocation hazards now eliminated from toy chests that comply with the standard. If in doubt about the safety of a storage box or bin, completely remove the lid. With the lid gone, your child cannot be trapped by it and cannot suffocate inside the box.

Many parents and caregivers use shelving to store toys. The greatest hazard with shelving occurs when a child pulls on it or tries to climb or stand on it. The shelving can tip over and crush the child. The key safety precaution with shelving, then, is to make sure the structure is attached securely to the wall or is designed so that it does not tip over.

Another challenge with toy storage—one that may test your ingenuity—is to try to keep toys intended for different age groups apart. Accomplishing this separation is crucial if you have older children as well as children younger than three years. Older children's toys often have small parts, small balls, and other components that are hazardous for younger children but not for the intended user. Here are some ways you may try to accomplish the challenging task of keeping children's toys separated:

- Get a different color storage box for each child.
- Designate a separate room for older children to store and play with their toys, and keep infants and toddlers away from this room.
- Explain to older children the importance of not letting their younger sibling play with small toys.

Swings, Slides, and Seesaws: Staying Safe at the Playground

Children adore playgrounds, where they can whiz through the air on a swing, whoosh down a slide, and clamber up climbing bars. Given this enthusiasm, there is little wonder that they can rush headlong into play equipment, slip from their footing, lose their handhold, or take a tumble. Incidents are bound to happen, but improved playground equipment, layout, and surfacing have helped to diminish them. The government and industry have made great progress in improving playground safety over the past decades. Guidelines and standards are in place for both public and home playgrounds. The standards are similar for the two settings, even though public playgrounds are maintained by a municipality or other entity while home playgrounds are the responsibility of parents and caregivers.

The public playground standard is a lengthy document that covers many types of equipment, including balance beams, climbers, upper body equipment, sliding poles, slides, swings, exercise rings/trapeze bars, moving/rotating/rocking components, seesaws, spring rockers, log rolls, and track rides. The standard addresses hazards from sharp points and edges, protrusions, pinch/crush/shear points, suspended hazards (cables, ropes, etc.), entrapment, entanglement, and falls. It also has requirements for structural integrity, surfacing, and access, including wheelchair access. No longer should you see equipment installed over asphalt, excessively high climbers, heavy swinging ride-on animals, very steep slides, wooden swing seats, and other serious hazards that were common on playgrounds in the 1950s and 1960s, and even into the 1970s. Today, you may even come across age-graded playgrounds. The layout of equipment at playgrounds usually allows a child's play to flow between the pieces with enough space for safe transition from one to the next.

The Americans with Disabilities Act requires that public playgrounds provide access for the disabled. The Access Board (www .access-board.gov) is the federal agency responsible for the development of design guidelines for accessibility. In the future, public playgrounds will need not only an access route but also opportunities for the disabled to play and interact with other children, both with and without disabilities, on types of equipment similar to the equipment the playground provides for children without disabilities.

Most playground injuries are associated with falls, and both public and home playground standards include requirements for protective surfaces to buffer those falls. Details about these protective surfaces, including what you should look for at public playgrounds and what you should install with backyard equipment, are given below in the section about injuries from falls.

Now that we've surveyed some of the general hazards associated with toys and playing—selecting appropriate toys, storing toys, and understanding playground settings—let's move on to specific injury hazards. In the following sections, I explain how to keep your child safe from the many hazards associated with indoor and outdoor toys and with playground equipment.

From Bruises to Broken Bones: Minimizing the Risk of Injury from Falls

As children toddle, run, and climb with no sense of danger, they are going to fall. When children walk, run, skate, and ride bicycles, tricycles, and scooters, they are going to fall. Whether children use backyard play equipment or the public playground, they are going to fall. They will fall as they race over the ground, as they pedal furiously into an object, and as they swing from one bar to the next on play equipment. Falls are going to happen, and they are going to happen repeatedly. Falls cause many injuries, ranging from minor bruises and cuts to broken bones, concussions, and death. You can minimize the severity of your child's injuries from falling if you take precautions with certain toys, have her use appropriate protective devices when biking or skating, and ensure that the play environment is "fall friendly."

Many injuries associated with toys are the result of a child's falling onto or off a toy or falling while carrying a toy, rather than the result of a child's playing as intended with a toy. A particularly serious injury—cuts on the roof of the mouth or the throat—can result when a child, typically a toddler, falls with an item in his mouth, especially if the item is tapered. Many reported incidents involve pencils or pens. Pencils and pens are not toys and should not be given to young children.

Since it is difficult to control the movements of a child, it is difficult to prevent falls. However, you can control the environment where a child might fall. Here are several examples of how you can control your child's play environment:

- Install an energy-absorbing surface beneath indoor climbing equipment. Carpets do not absorb energy. If you don't have a truly energy-absorbing surface, don't have the climbing equipment.
- Limit other types of indoor play to an area that is carpeted to reduce the risk of children's sliding and falling.
- Barricade stairs with a gate. (Gates are marketed as either *for* or *not for* use at the top of stairs. Never use a "not for top of stairs" gate at the top of a flight of stairs.)
- Ensure that furniture in a child's play area is made of unbreakable material and does not have sharp edges.
- Encourage children to put their toys away after play sessions.

- Restrict outdoor play to certain approved areas where there is adequate protective surfacing and where motor vehicles are not allowed.

Falls from a height are more dangerous than falls at ground level, because they generate more energy. Higher levels of energy always have the potential for more serious injury. The only way to minimize injury is to have something other than a child's body absorb that energy.

Falls from a height frequently occur with playground equipment. The industry standard states that home playground equipment must come with instructions about protective surfacing materials. Protective surfaces are intended to absorb most of the energy associated with a fall, so that a child's body absorbs as little energy as possible on impact. If the child absorbs too much energy, he will be injured. When you buy home play equipment, the user's manual and other accompanying literature will suggest protective materials and their appropriate depth. Note that grass does not count as a protective surface, because immediately underneath the layer of grass lies compact ground, which is both hard and unyielding. You should install backyard equipment over shredded mulch, wood chips, fine gravel, or fine sand to the depth recommended by the equipment manufacturer. Routinely inspect the protective surface, because you will need to replace, replenish, or redistribute it to maintain the recommended depth and condition. Another protective surface that you may see at a public playground or want to use at home is synthetic surfacing sold in individual units. Examples of synthetic surfacing are rubber mats,

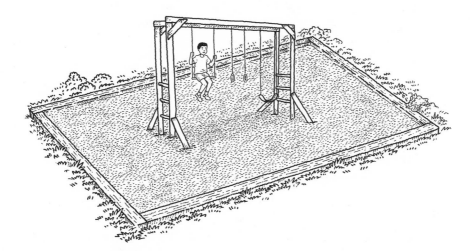

rubber tiles, and poured-in-place materials. Compared to loose-fill materials, synthetic unit surfacing requires little maintenance, but it is more expensive to install initially.

The industry standard for public playground equipment requires that the owner or operator install and maintain appropriate protective surfacing. For the most part, playground operators install the required surfacing, but they often fall short on maintenance. Typical protective surfaces become worn with use and weather, resulting in thin or bare spots (especially around slides and swings) and areas where the surface has become compact. These kinds of changes in the protective surface alter its ability to perform correctly, and therefore falls onto these compromised surfaces are more likely to result in injury. If you see playground surfaces that concern you, report them to the municipality or other entity responsible for public playground maintenance and insist that the surfacing be brought back to adequate levels.

Like falls from heights, falls from bikes, scooters, skates, and other moving items produce higher energy. The higher energy results from greater speed and increases the potential for serious injury. To minimize injury, something other than the child's body must absorb the energy. Helmets, knee pads, and elbow pads are the best items for a child to wear for these activities. Get your child into the habit of always wearing a helmet on her bike, scooter, or skates, and make sure that she wears it correctly. There are many types of retention systems on helmets, and it is very important to read and understand the fit instructions and warnings contained in the manual that came with the helmet. Severe head injuries and death can result from the impact of hitting a street surface or colliding with a motor vehicle. A helmet is intended to absorb much of the energy from an impact and can make a life-saving difference for your child.

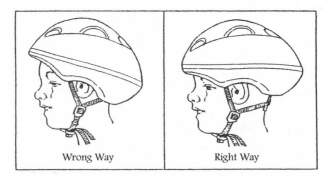

Wrong Way   Right Way

✦ Key Actions to Prevent Injury from Falls

You can reduce the likelihood of your child's being badly injured from a fall in the following ways.

1. Soften the fall environment indoors by minimizing exposure to sharp edges on furniture and to breakables and by having a proper protective surface under climbing equipment.
2. Soften the fall environment outdoors by having a truly protective surface, not just grass, beneath backyard play equipment.
3. Insist that proper surfaces be installed and maintained at public playgrounds.
4. Get your child in the habit of wearing a helmet and other protective equipment while riding bikes or scooters and while skating.
5. Make sure protective equipment, especially a helmet, is worn correctly, according to the manufacturer's instructions.
6. Have your child put away his toys when playtime is over.
7. If your child plays with toys intended to go in the mouth, such as musical instruments, have her remain seated while using the toys, especially if she is younger than two years.

Loose Strings: What Causes Tangling, Hanging, and Strangling Incidents?

The clothing your child wears to play can be as important to safety as the toys or equipment with which he plays. You may have noticed that children's outerwear—sweatshirts and jackets—no longer has drawstrings at the neck. Even if you wanted to buy a child's garment with a drawstring hood or neck cuff, you wouldn't find one, because an industry standard went into effect in 1997 prohibiting the sale of outerwear in sizes 2T to 12 with drawstrings at the neck. If you come across children's outerwear with drawstrings at the neck at a second-hand store or yard sale, tell the seller to either remove the drawstrings or not sell or donate the item.

The standard came about because of several hanging deaths and near-misses, especially on playground slides, after clothing drawstrings got snagged in the equipment. Children at highest risk were five to eight years old. Typically, the neckline drawstring caught in a

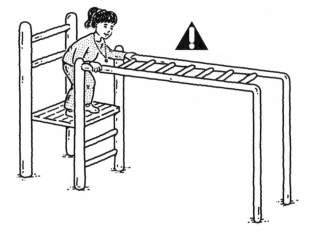

V-opening near the top of the slide, and as the child came down the slide, the drawstring pulled taut so that the jacket tightened at the neck and the child hung. Scarves and necklaces can be similarly dangerous when they catch on protrusions.

Just as strings on clothing are hazards, so too are strings on toys themselves. When you see a toy with a string, ribbon, cord, or rope, you should immediately think of the danger of a child's being tangled in it or strangled by it. A string that is long and loose on one end can easily wrap around a child's neck or another body part. Years ago, when toy telephones were made with long, stretchy cords, toddlers inevitably got tangled up in them. In the early 1990s, a one-year-old boy got the string of a toy car wrapped around his neck, and he was strangled. Children younger than eighteen months can roll in and get wrapped in cords, but they cannot get untangled by themselves. Today, the toy safety standard limits the length of cords on toys intended for children younger than eighteen months to less than 12 inches. The one exception is pull toys, which are allowed to have longer strings for practical reasons. However, the end of the string on a pull toy must not have knots, loops, beads, or other items, because these could get caught on another part of the toy and form a loop large enough for a child's head to enter. To keep your child safe, do not alter strings or add strings to toys beyond what comes with them at purchase.

As discussed earlier in this chapter and in Chapter 2, toys intended to be strung across a crib or tied to side rails or end rails (for example, crib gyms and activity centers) pose a strangling hazard, since an infant can fall across the suspended item and strangle from the weight of her head (see illustration on p. 33). Crib mobiles typically have figures suspended by string, and when children are able to reach high enough, these strings can become wound around fingers and cut off the blood supply. A child should be able to see a crib mobile but not reach it. In one instance, a standing child's bib got caught on a screw attaching a mobile to a crib; had the mother not found her child, now trapped at the neckline, the child could have strangled or hung. Labels on crib gyms and crib mobiles recommend removing these products from the crib when a baby reaches five months. By this age, a child is pushing up with his hands and legs, and although he probably isn't yet pulling to a standing position, which is particularly problematic with mobiles, the mobile label recommendation adds a safety buffer. When you remove the crib gym, remove the mobile as well and hang these items on a wall, out of reach.

Strings and cords also cause problems for older children. In 2003, several incidents occurred with water yo-yos, which are water-filled balls on the end of an elasticized string. Children, mostly five years and older, got the string wrapped around their neck. Fortunately, none of them were strangled. The New York Consumer Protection Board asked stores throughout New York State to pull the water yo-yos from their shelves, and the state of Illinois banned them outright. A bill proposed in the U.S. Congress would direct the Consumer Product Safety Commission to declare a national ban on water yo-yos. Several other countries have already banned these toys.

Bike helmet straps also pose a strangling or hanging hazard when a child wears her helmet to play on playground equipment, because the straps can snag on protrusions. Teach your child to remove her helmet while on playground equipment—and to put it back on when she leaves on her bike or skates.

⚓ Key Actions to Prevent Tangling, Hanging, and Strangling Injuries

There are several ways you can keep your child safe from tangling, hanging, and strangling injuries.

1. Let your child play in comfortable clothing without any type of strings, ribbons, or cords attached, especially at the neckline.
2. Do not let your child wear anything looped around his neck, such as play binoculars or a necklace, when he goes to the playground.
3. Never add strings or cords to toys.
4. Remove crib toys (mobiles and gyms) when your baby reaches five months old.
5. Have your child remove her bike helmet before playing on playground equipment.

Small Spaces: How to Prevent Your Child
from Becoming Trapped

Children enjoy getting into small spaces where adults can't go. The danger of small spaces, though, is that children can easily be trapped and unable to free themselves. A child generally becomes trapped in one of three ways:

1. A child gets into a space that is large enough for part of his body to pass through but not large enough for his entire body. Usually, the head—the largest body part—gets stuck.
2. A child is inside something that collapses and traps her. For example, a collapsed playpen can trap a child inside.
3. A child enters an unventilated space and pulls a lid or door closed.

In all three of these trapping scenarios, suffocation and strangling are the most severe possible outcomes.

In the first scenario, a child does not realize that different parts of his body are different sizes and shapes. It doesn't even occur to him that after he fits one part of his body through an opening, the rest may not follow as easily. A child enters a space either head first or foot first. The head varies in its dimensions—for example, head width is fairly small, head height is larger, and head length is larger still. The dimensions shown in the illustration are average for children thirty-one to thirty-six months old. The head can also be oriented in differ-

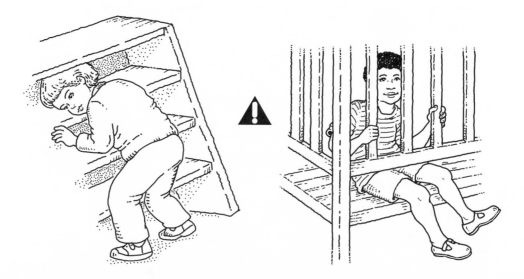

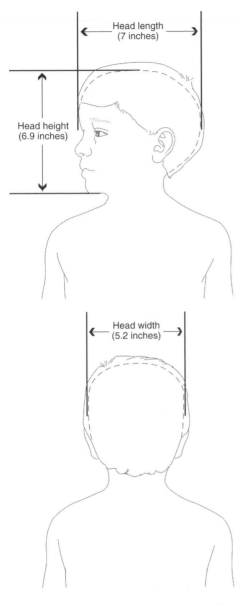

Head length
(7 inches)

Head height
(6.9 inches)

Head width
(5.2 inches)

ent ways. It can be manipulated to fit into smallish openings in one orientation, perhaps one that allows head width to enter. Once the head has passed through an opening, a person's normal tendency is to right his head. However, if the space was just large enough for the head width, it will be too small for the head height. In this situation, a child cannot figure out how to reorient his head to back out of the opening, and he can panic or freeze. A child trapped by the head can die from strangling if there is pressure on the neck.

Foot-first trapping occurs because the lower torso (from the hips down) fits into a much narrower space than does the upper torso (chest and shoulders) and head. When gravity takes over and a child falls into the space she put her feet into, she can be trapped either by her chest and shoulders or by her head. In either case, she can suffocate or strangle.

The openings on playground equipment are specifically designed to prevent both head-first and foot-first trapping. Playground equipment that meets the ASTM standard should not pose any trapping hazard. Spaces that are wide enough to allow a child's hips to fit through (3½ inches or wider) must also be large enough to allow the head to pass through (9 inches). So openings should be either smaller than 3½ inches or larger than 9 inches, but not in between. In the previous section, I mentioned that a child wearing a bike helmet may become tangled in playground equipment; another reason to remove a bike helmet on the playground is that helmets, in effect, increase the size of a child's head and can cause trapping incidents.

The second trapping scenario listed above involves an item collapsing on a child who is inside it (see illustration on p. 34). Any product that folds, such as a playpen or a walker, has the potential to fold unexpectedly and trap a child. Depending on how the child is trapped, the possible consequences include suffocation and strangling. Several brands of playpen sold in the 1990s were recalled by the Consumer Product Safety Commission, which had been alerted to at least fourteen suffocation or strangling deaths associated with their collapse. If you have a folding product with locking latches, follow all instructions to ensure that the locks are secure. If products fold in spite of their locking mechanism, stop using them and report them to the manufacturer and to the Consumer Product Safety Commission.

The third trapping scenario arises from a child's curiosity and play behavior. Climbing into spaces and looking for places to hide are normal activities, whether the space be a car trunk, a toy chest, a hope chest, a closet, or some other enclosure. Spaces that have the potential to close, or worse, to lock, present a risk of suffocation. Discarded refrigerators used to be notorious suffocation hazards. When children get into closed spaces, they may lack either the strength required to open the closure or the cognitive skill to figure out how to escape.

An industry safety standard addresses lid closures and ventilation holes in toy chests, and the Refrigerator Safety Act requires that it be possible to open a refrigerator from the inside. However, many other places in which children get trapped are not subject to any safety standards that specifically address the risk of childhood suffocation. This means that you must be vigilant and recognize such hazards. The most unusual product I have come across that was involved in a trapping death was a cooler. A little boy climbed into the cooler while at a family picnic; no one noticed, and no one thought to look for him in the cooler.

❦ Key Actions to Prevent Trapping Incidents

You can do several things to reduce the risk of your child's becoming trapped.

1. Check that your home playground equipment indicates compliance with ASTM F 1148. As of this book's publication, the latest version was published in 2003. If you are unsure, contact the manufacturer.
2. Check that your public playground equipment complies with ASTM F 1487. As of this book's publication, the latest ver-

sion was published in 2005. If you are unsure, ask the municipality or other entity responsible for the playground.

3. If there is no record that a public playground has been tested for adherence to the ASTM standard, ask that a certified playground safety inspector be hired. The National Playground Safety Institute's website (www.nrpa.org) has a link to qualified contractors (www.playground-contractors.org). In addition, the National Program for Playground Safety (1-800-554-PLAY; www.playgroundsafety.org or www.uni.edu/playground) may be able to answer your questions.

4. Have your child remove his bike helmet before playing on playground equipment.

5. Make sure toy chests either do not have a lid or have one that meets the industry standard—that is, a lid with special hinges to prevent complete and sudden closing.

6. Be aware that spaces large enough for children to climb into must be ventilated. Keep vehicles, hope chests, and other unventilated enclosures locked or otherwise inaccessible to children.

Blocked Airway: Knowing How to Avoid Choking Hazards

From the time children have the skill to reach for and pick up objects, they will put any sort of object they find into their mouth. Children have no concept of which objects may be hazardous to them, so into the mouth goes everything from building blocks to books to balloons. Although children most commonly choke on food, they can also choke on the small parts of toys, small balls, marbles, and balloons. Small items such as these are a hazard, especially for children younger than three years, but for older children as well. For example, a five-year-old Wisconsin boy died after inhaling a fragment of a burst helium-inflated latex balloon that was left from a party; a six-year-old Texas girl choked on a small rubber ball given away as a promotion by a fast-food restaurant.

The federal mandatory regulation, which came into effect in 1979, does not allow small parts to be accessible in toys and articles intended for children younger than three years old. The regulation uses a truncated cylinder of a specific shape and size to determine whether an item is technically a small part. The cylinder has a diameter of 1¼ inches and a depth varying from 1 to 2¼ inches. Any item that

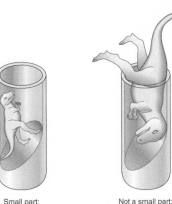

Small part:
fits totally inside cylinder

Not a small part:
does not fit totally inside cylinder

fits completely within it is considered a small part. If you would like to test toys or other items at home, you can buy a small-parts test cylinder from toy stores, children's furniture and accessories stores, and stores that specialize in child safety, or you may find one free at a booth at a safety fair. Some people recommend using a cardboard toilet-paper roll as a substitute, even though it has a larger opening and much greater depth than the actual test cylinder. If you use a toilet-paper roll, you will at least err on the side of safety—while some items that fit into the roll will not actually be small parts, you can be certain that all items that technically are small parts will fit into it.

The regulation ensures that most products intended for children younger than three years are free of small parts when the product is assembled, but it does not automatically mean that all products are in compliance. Each year, the Consumer Product Safety Commission recalls many products that violate the small parts regulation. In other cases, they recall a product because it breaks and creates or releases a small part.

Latex balloons must be labeled, as mentioned in the list of toy labels near the beginning of this chapter, to inform caregivers about the choking hazard. Broken and uninflated latex balloons are responsible for more choking deaths in the first year of life than any other non-food item. Remember that inflated balloons are not the problem; only broken and uninflated balloons are. Be extremely vigilant when your children are around latex balloons, and immediately discard the pieces of a broken balloon. Mylar® balloons are a good alternative, because they do not pose the choking hazard that latex balloons do. Mylar® doesn't break and doesn't conform to the throat.

Round and conical shapes are the worst offenders for choking incidents (just as they are with foods), because they can lodge snugly at the back of the throat and be very difficult to extract. Since the small parts requirement came into effect in 1979, evidence has surfaced that rounded items as large as 1¾ inches in diameter—too large to be considered small parts—can be choking hazards. For this reason, small balls (defined as those with a diameter less than 1¾ inches) must be labeled as not for children younger than three years. In addition, small balls included as part of a toy or game for children aged three to eight must be labeled as not for children younger than three.

By federal regulation, rattles must also be too large to enter a child's mouth and block the back of the throat. Rattles are tested with an oval template. In order to comply with the regulation, no part of a rattle can go through to the full depth of the template; if it does, the rattle violates the regulation and the Consumer Product Safety Commission has the authority to ban it. Squeeze toys can present a hazard similar to rattles and should, in their noncompressed state, also be too large to reach the back of a child's throat. As part of the industry toy standard, squeeze toys are tested with the same depth criterion as rattles, using a modified rattle template with a diameter of 1.68 (about $1^{11}/_{16}$) inches.

There is a relatively new phenomenon that I'd like to bring to your attention before leaving the subject of choking. As mentioned in Chapter 4, sometimes children swallow items, and although that's not technically choking, it can still be serious. Normally, if a small part is swallowed and makes its way to the stomach, it passes without harm in the child's bowel movement. In 2005, a toddler swallowed several tiny but powerful magnets from a toy that belonged to his older brother. Once the magnets were in his intestine, they exerted a powerful attraction on one another, and in moving toward one another they distorted and obstructed his intestine. The child became ill with flulike symptoms and died in the hospital. Only after an autopsy was performed did anyone realize what had happened.

According to press release 06-127, issued in March 2006, the Consumer Product Safety Commission is aware of thirty-four incidents involving small magnets, including the above-mentioned death and four serious injuries. Among the serious injuries, three children in the age range of three to eight years had intestinal perforations that required surgery and hospitalization in intensive care, and a five-year-old child aspirated two magnets that were surgically removed from his lung. If you purchase a toy that contains magnets, examine the toy regularly to make sure that the toy remains intact and no magnets are released.

ʅ Key Actions to Prevent Choking on Toys

Reduce the chance that your child will put a small object into his mouth and be at risk of choking.

  1. Keep small balls, marbles, and toys with small parts away

from children, especially children younger than three years old, because they like to put objects into their mouth.

2. Assemble toys that have small parts (screws, batteries, etc.) when children younger than three years are not in the same room and are not watching you.

3. Do not allow a child younger than eight years old to blow up a balloon. Instead, you should blow the balloon up for the child.

4. Discard broken balloons immediately. Uninflated and broken latex balloons present serious choking hazards.

5. If you purchase a toy that contains magnets, examine the toy regularly to make sure that the toy remains intact and no magnets are released.

No Air: Recognizing Suffocation Hazards

Mechanical suffocation—suffocating because an object has covered the nose and mouth, or as a result of chest compression—usually happens in the first year of life and is most common in a child's sleep environment rather than her play environment. However, an unusual 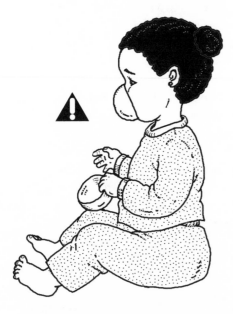 situation arises with toys that are cup-, oval-, and half-egg-shaped containers. Children have placed a hollowed-out half over their nose and mouth, and the container has become stuck in place by a strong suction force. This force tends to be so strong that without adult intervention the child can suffocate. Although many years ago a few such incidents occurred with L'Eggs pantyhose containers, people's attention became focused on this hazard in 1999, when Pokemon balls given out in children's meals by Burger King caused at least two deaths. Pokemon balls were plastic ball-shaped containers between 2¾ and 3 inches in diameter. The two halves of the container pulled apart to reveal a toy. A four-month-old boy in Indianapolis suffocated when one half of a Pokemon ball, which was in his crib, became stuck on his face. Then a thirteen-month-old girl suffocated when half of a Pokemon ball covered her nose and mouth. An eighteen-month-old girl nearly suffocated when half of a Pokemon ball got stuck over her face, but fortunately, on his second attempt the girl's father was able to pull it off her face.

The packaging that accompanied Pokemon balls described them as safety tested and recommended for children of all ages; this illustrates how a product can pass a safety test yet still be hazardous. When the Pokemon balls were tested, the toy standard did not address the hazard of hollow shapes, so manufacturers had no way to test this aspect of the toy. Now the standard has an updated section that refers specifically to this hazard.

Finally, remember that thin plastic bags and plastic wrappings are always a cause for concern, especially with children younger than one year old. If toys (or any other item, such as magazines, groceries, etc.) are packaged in plastic or plastic bags, discard the plastic immediately.

Key Actions to Prevent Suffocation

You can avoid situations where your child is at risk of suffocating by keeping these hazards in mind.

1. Keep thin plastic away from children, especially children younger than one year old.
2. Keep hollowed-out, lightweight containers with a diameter of 2½ to 4 inches away from young children, especially children younger than three years old.

Watch Your Fingers! What Causes Pinching, Crushing, and Shearing?

The point of contact between two moving parts can pinch, crush, or shear a body part that gets in between these moving parts. Usually it is fingers that suffer this type of injury; fingertip amputation is an example of a severe outcome. Toys and play equipment designed to comply with ASTM standards do not have moving parts that create pinch, crush, or shear hazards. Nonetheless, these hazards still occur in some products: children's folding chairs, for instance, can suddenly collapse, or a child can get her finger caught in one of them while folding or unfolding it.

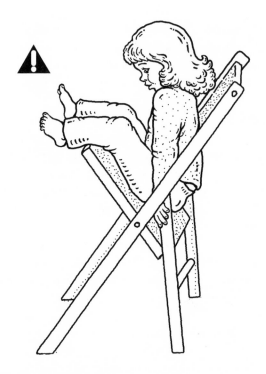

❦ Key Actions to Prevent Pinching, Crushing, and Shearing

To minimize the chance that your child's fingers or other body parts will be pinched, crushed, or sheared, make sure that folding toys and other products, especially those designed to bear a child's weight, are in the fully locked position when set up.

Being Cool: Avoiding Burns during Playtime

One of the nicest things about outdoor play is the warmth and brightness of the sun. It just seems that everyone is happier in the sun. But sunburn is a serious matter—sunburns hurt and can cause dehydration and fever—and exposure to the sun's rays is a cause of skin cancer. Although skin cancer is rare among children, its prevalence in older adults speaks to the cumulative effect of sun exposure. According to the American Academy of Pediatrics, our skin "remembers" every sunburn. Having one or more blistering sunburns as a child increases the risk of developing skin cancer later in life.

Since children spend a lot of time playing outdoors, especially in the summer months, it is important to protect them from the damaging rays of the sun. A combination of limiting time outdoors, wearing protective clothing, and putting on sunscreen is a proven way to reduce the risks. Babies younger than six months old need special protection, because their skin is thinner and more sensitive than even an older child's skin is. Even babies with naturally darker skin need special protection. As indicated in the American Academy of Pediatrics recommendations listed below, sunscreen may not be appropriate for babies younger than six months.

Sunscreens are regulated by the Food and Drug Administration (FDA). Sunscreens are labeled with SPF numbers. SPF stands for "sun protection factor." The higher the SPF number, the more sunburn protection the product provides. *Sunscreen alone is not enough, however.* In fact, using sunscreen often lulls people into the mistaken assumption that they are protected from all of the sun's damaging rays. This is not true. Much more effective than sunscreen alone is sunscreen along with hats, long sleeves, cover-ups, sun umbrellas and staying out of the sun completely between the hours of 10:00 a.m. and 4:00 p.m. For sunscreens to work, they must be applied in adequate amounts. Be mindful that sunscreen can wash off, be rubbed off, or sweat off. So you probably need to apply sunscreen liberally and more than once in a single outing.

The FDA is concerned about the health hazards associated with suntanning products that do not contain sunscreen ingredients. Beginning May 22, 2000, such suntanning products must bear the following: "*Warning*—This product does not contain a sunscreen and does not protect against sunburn. Repeated exposure of unprotected skin while tanning may increase the risk of skin aging, skin cancer, and other harmful effects to the skin even if you do not burn."

Your children younger than one can enjoy the outdoors and stay protected from the harmful rays of the sun if you follow these recommendations from the American Academy of Pediatrics (AAP):

- Keep babies younger than 6 months old out of direct sunlight. Move your baby to the shade or under a tree, umbrella or the stroller canopy.
- Dress your baby in clothing that covers the body, such as comfortable lightweight long pants, long-sleeved shirts, and hats with brims that shade the face and cover the ears.
- If your baby gets a sunburn and is younger than 1 year of age, contact your pediatrician at once; a severe sunburn is an emergency.

- For babies younger than 6 months of age, the risks or benefits of sunscreen use are not yet known. If your baby needs to be outdoors, discuss sunscreen use and other options with your pediatrician.
- For babies older than 6 months of age, choose a sunscreen made for children.

Follow these AAP recommendations for your children older than one:

- Choose a sunscreen that is made for children, preferably waterproof. Before covering your child completely, test the sunscreen on your child's back for a reaction. Apply carefully around the eyes, avoiding the eyelids. If a rash develops, talk to your pediatrician.
- Select clothes made of tightly woven fabrics. Clothes that have a tighter weave—that is, the way a fabric is constructed—generally protect better than clothes with a broader weave. If you're not sure about how tight a fabric's weave is, hold the clothing up to a lamp or window and see how much light shines through. The less light, the better. Clothing made of cotton is both cool and protective.
- When using a cap with a bill (like a baseball cap), make sure the bill is facing forward to shield your child's face. Sunglasses with UV protection also are a good idea for protecting your child's eyes. Play sunglasses do not offer the protection of real sunglasses.
- If your child gets a sunburn that results in blistering, pain or fever, contact your pediatrician.

The AAP offers further sun safety tips for all members of your family:

- Try to keep out of the sun between the hours of 10 a.m. and 4 p.m. because the sun's rays are the strongest then.
- The sun's damaging UV rays can bounce back from sand, snow, water or concrete, so be particularly careful in these areas.
- Most of the sun's rays can come through the clouds on an overcast day, so use sun protection even on cloudy days. When choosing a sunscreen, look for the words "broad-spectrum" on the label; those words mean that the sunscreen will screen out both ultraviolet B (UVB) and ultraviolet A (UVA) rays. Sunburn is associated with ultraviolet B (UVB); ultraviolet A

(UVA), however, can penetrate the skin and damage connective tissue at deeper levels, even if the skin's surface feels cool. It is important to limit exposure to both UVA and UVB.

- Choose a water-resistant or waterproof sunscreen. Sunscreens that are "waterproof" should be reapplied every two hours, especially if your child is playing in the water.
- Zinc oxide, a very effective sunblock, can be used as extra protection on the nose, cheeks, tops of the ears and on the shoulders.
- Use a sun protection factor (SPF) of at least 15.
- Rub sunscreen in well, making sure to cover all exposed areas, especially your child's face, nose, ears, feet and hands, and even the backs of the knees.
- Put on sunscreen 30 minutes before going outdoors—it needs time to work on the skin.
- If your child does get sunburned, keep her completely out of the sun until the sunburn is totally healed.
- Sunscreens should be used for sun protection and not as a reason to stay in the sun longer.

The sun also heats up other surfaces outside. When a child touches a hot surface, even for a brief moment, he can be injured with a thermal or contact burn. Metal, plastic, and concrete surfaces can become hot from the sun—for example, think of playground equipment in direct sunlight. Surfaces can also become hot from heat generated within a toy, usually a battery-operated toy. If you leave batteries in a product for a long time without using it, insert batteries incorrectly, or mix battery types, the batteries may overheat, leak, or explode. A child who comes into contact with the substance that leaks out from batteries can suffer a chemical burn.

⌁ Key Actions to Prevent Burns

Keep your child safe from burns during playtime by following AAP guidelines, above, and with the following actions.

1. Position backyard play equipment with the sun's path in mind. Plant bushes or trees to provide shade.
2. Before children use play equipment, touch the surfaces, especially of slides, to make sure they are not hot from the sun.
3. Monitor the use of battery-operated toys, and make sure that

you use the recommended type and size of battery, install batteries in the correct orientation, and replace all batteries at the same time when one or more appears weak.

What Did You Say? Preventing Hearing Damage

Most of us take our hearing for granted, but hearing impairment and hearing loss affect many people all over the world. Several studies have shown that long-term hearing loss occurs when a person is exposed to loud sounds. As of 2003, a section of the toy standard addresses acceptable sound levels for toys. Sound levels are measured in decibels, with a higher decibel, or dB, indicating a louder sound. To minimize the risk of your child's experiencing hearing damage, choose toys with tones that are soft and soothing, and never place the source of a noise close to your child's ear. Although listening to music on a Walkman-style unit or a digital audio player is probably more of an issue for older children, it's worth mentioning. Several styles of headphone deliver music straight into the ear canal and, along with high music volume, can cause long-term hearing loss. Digital audio players may pose an additional risk beyond that of Walkman-style units, because digital players store hundreds of songs and play continuously. To minimize the risk from these products, pay attention to the volume at which your child listens to music and the length of time he listens for.

Key Actions to Prevent Hearing Damage

You can avoid situations where your child would be at risk of hearing damage.

1. Avoid toys that make loud, impulsive noises. Impulsive noises can be short and explosive (the sound rises quickly and lasts only a brief time) or extended (the sound rises more slowly and lasts longer than an explosion).
2. Do not hold noise-producing toys close to your child's ear.
3. Monitor the volume and the length of time your child spends listening to music through headphones.

Summing Up

Playtime is a significant part of the day for any child, no matter her age, ability, or interests. As with any activity, a child's play environment and the toys and equipment he plays with pose certain hazards. It wasn't possible to address every known playtime injury and scenario in this chapter. However, I have described some common injuries and injury circumstances (such as playground falls) as well as less common injuries and situations (such as hanging on a crib gym), all of which can result in severe injury or death. The key for parents and caregivers is to carefully monitor their children's play behavior and environment without diminishing the creative fun that will keep their children growing and learning.

Play Safely Checklist

The following Play Safely Checklist has three parts: indoor play, outdoor play, and general play. Go through the checklist as you consider your child's play behavior and environment.

Indoor Play

1. Do you read and use age-grade information before buying toys for your child?

   Manufacturers use age grading to indicate the appropriate general age for which their product is intended. Age grading considers a typical child's abilities and the related safety issues for the child's age group. Safety tests are performed on toys according to the age grading.

2. Once you bring toys home, do you keep your older children's toys away from your younger children?

   There are different safety issues for different age groups. Some toys that are safe for certain age groups present a risk of injury for other age groups. Exercise care in keeping toys separate, especially toys that indicate a hazard for a younger user.

3. Where are your children's toys stored? Are there trapping hazards (such as a heavy lid that does not stay open) or compression hazards (such as shelving that is not secured to the wall and tends to tip forward)?

Children want to be able to reach their toys, whether the toys are in a bin or a box or are up on a shelf. Make sure that bin and box lids have been removed or have a mechanism to keep them from dropping closed. Make sure that shelving is securely attached to the wall.

4. Does your child put away her toys after playtime?

Children are often injured when they trip over toys on the floor, on stairways, and elsewhere. Encourage children to put away toys after play.

5. Are designated inside play areas free of sharp corners (such as the corners on coffee tables), glass furniture, and breakables? Are play areas carpeted?

Children, and especially toddlers, inevitably fall when they play, so try to make their play spaces as "fall friendly" as possible. If you have indoor climbing equipment for your child, you should have a mat that meets safe surfacing requirements under and around it.

6. Are you aware of the choking hazard presented by balloons, small balls, and marbles?

These items are extremely hazardous to children. Blow up all latex balloons for children younger than eight years, and throw away broken balloons immediately. Keep small balls away from children younger than four years, even though small balls are considered acceptable for children three and older. I recommend keeping marbles away from children until they are older than five years, despite manufacturers' age grading of three years and older.

7. Have you removed crib gyms and mobiles from the crib by the time your child can push up on his hands and knees at about age five months?

Crib gyms and mobiles are intended as visual toys. They can present strangling and tangling hazards when they are within an infant's reach. Be sure to remove them from the crib by the time your infant is five months old.

Outdoor Play

1. How is your child dressed for play?

Remember that drawstrings, scarves, and any item looped

around the neck (for example, a necklace or a toy camera on a strap) easily catch on protrusions or snag in openings. Playground equipment that does not comply with ASTM's protrusion requirements poses particularly serious hazards when children wear clothes or items with strings near the neck. Ensure that your child wears comfortable clothing without any string, ribbon, loop, or loose flowing material attached.

2. Does your child wear appropriate protective items when she uses a bike, scooter, or other product with wheels?

    Helmets are essential as soon as a child begins to ride a bike or rides as a passenger on your bike. Be sure to follow the manufacturer's instructions for proper fit and adjustment of the helmet. In addition, knee and elbow pads help to minimize injuries when a child uses skates and scooters.

3. Have you taught your child to remove his bike helmet before playing on playground equipment?

    Bike helmet straps can get caught on playground equipment. In addition, the helmet increases the size of your child's head, so trapping becomes a possibility. Teach your child that helmets are essential for bike riding but must be removed for playground play.

4. Is the surface under playground equipment protective?

    Protective surfacing absorbs the energy from falls so that a child's body does not absorb that energy and, in the process, get injured. Grass is not a protective surface, because underneath it is packed, hard ground. The required depth of the protective surface depends on the height of the equipment and the type of surfacing you select. Loose-fill protective surfacing, such as wood chips and sand, needs to be replenished and redistributed regularly.

5. Have you taken measures to protect your child from sunburn?

    Sunburn is serious, and the sun's ultraviolet rays can cause cancer later in life. A combination of three strategies works best: apply sunscreen to children older than six months, have children wear protective clothing, like brimmed hats and long sleeves, and limit their time outdoors, especially between 10:00 a.m. and 4:00 p.m.

General Play

1. With battery-operated toys, do you ensure that batteries are fresh, are all of the same type and size, and are inserted in the correct orientation?

   Batteries can leak, overheat, or explode if they are mixed (that is, mixed types of battery or mixed old and new batteries), inserted incorrectly, or left in toys that are not used for long periods.

2. Do you check that any foldable item (like a playpen or chair) used by your child is in its fully locked position prior to use?

   When products unintentionally collapse, they can create trapping, pinching, shearing, crushing, and amputation hazards.

3. Do you discard any thin plastic packaging right away, especially if your child is younger than one year?

   Infants can suffocate on thin plastic. Discard packaging, wrapping, and plastic bags immediately after opening products.

4. Are you aware that loud, impulsive noises can cause hearing damage in children of all ages?

   Avoid toys that make very loud sounds. Do not put noise-making toys close to your child's ears.

6

🌸 Are We There Yet?

Traveling Near and Far

Most of us travel somewhere every day, whether on foot, on a bike, by bus, or in a car. With an infant or child in tow, travel becomes a little more complex, but most children love to go places, even if you are taking them only as far as the grocery store.

No matter where you go and how you get there, you need to think about the safest way to take your child. In a vehicle, car seats and booster seats are absolute necessities. On foot with a stroller or carriage, safety restraints and wheel locks help keep your child safe. Even while you "travel" around the grocery store with a shopping cart, there are safety concerns to keep in mind.

Driving down the Street: Injury from Motor Vehicles

Motor vehicle crashes claim more children's lives each year than do any other kinds of unintentional injury. Vehicle crashes will probably always remain at the top of the list, because the energy created by moving vehicles is tremendous—and (as I explained earlier) injury depends on the amount of energy absorbed by the body. A vehicle's energy is related to its weight and the speed at which it travels. When a vehicle comes to a sudden stop or crashes, some of its energy transfers to the passengers inside. An unrestrained child (or adult, for that matter) could be thrown around inside the vehicle or could be thrown out of it. Every single U.S. state requires children to be buckled up.

When a vehicle rolls over, the potential to be thrown around inside or thrown outside it naturally increases. According to the Coalition for Consumer Health and Safety, light trucks, minivans, vans, and sport utility vehicles (SUVs) are much more susceptible than cars to flipping over on sharp turns, at corners, and when the driver attempts a quick maneuver. These types of vehicle roll over so easily because they sit up high and do not hug the road as cars do. Consider this roll-over potential when you choose a vehicle.

Crashes and roll-overs are not the only types of injury incident that occur with vehicles. Parents have run over their children in their own driveway. Before backing out of a driveway, make sure you can account for all children who may be nearby, and don't forget that your neighbors' children may be around too. Young children cannot be seen behind a vehicle, so walk around your vehicle to check before driving. Some newer cars are equipped with technology sensors that alert the driver if her reversing car is approaching an object too closely.

If you stop to run an errand, do not leave children alone in the car. Children have died from hyperthermia (excessive heat) when left in a vehicle with the windows up in hot weather. Children have also started cars with keys in the ignition, have strangled when their clothing caught on a turn signal, have strangled on the harness as they struggled to get out of their car seat, and have trapped themselves in automatic windows.

Also remember that vehicle engines produce carbon monoxide, an odorless and colorless poisonous gas. When you drive down the street, carbon monoxide is not a problem for the vehicle's occupants, because it dissipates into the air. However, if the engine runs in an enclosed space, carbon monoxide builds up to dangerous levels. To prevent carbon monoxide poisoning, never start or run a vehicle in a closed garage, and never leave a child in a vehicle with the engine running, because the carbon monoxide can accumulate and enter the vehicle.

Strapped In: Car Seats, Booster Seats, and Seat Belts

When most of us get into a car, we put on the seat belt—it's second nature. But young children need to have their seat belt or other restraint system secured for them, and older children may need to be reminded about buckling up. A 2005 study showed that inappropriately restrained children were about twice as likely to be injured as appropriately restrained children.

As well as being correctly buckled in, it matters where a child sits in a vehicle. The same study found that unrestrained children in the front seat were at highest risk of injury, while appropriately restrained children in the rear seat were at lowest risk.

Car safety seats and seat belts are intended to protect a child, especially in the case of a head-on collision. Their role is to keep the child in position and to absorb much of the energy generated during a crash or an abrupt stop. Buying a car seat may be the easiest part of the process. Correctly installing and using the seat may be more difficult, but it is essential that you install and use a car seat properly to keep your child as safe as possible. Car seat checks, conducted by organizations like Safe Kids, have repeatedly shown that most car seats are not doing the job they're designed to do, because either the seat is not properly secured in the vehicle or the child is not properly restrained within the seat. A 2005 study from several states showed that car seats are misused 73 percent of the time. Most commonly, harness straps are too loose on the child, and the vehicle's seat belt is attached too loosely to the car seat. Unless the car seat is installed correctly and the child is buckled in correctly, the seat may not protect the child in a crash.

If a car seat check event is held in your community, drive through and have the staff check out your seat installation. A Maryland mother who did this at a Safe Kids car check event had both of her children's seats adjusted. Later the same day, she was involved in a crash, and her children were uninjured.

Most new vehicles now have a standardized attachment system to simplify car seat installation and to enhance safety. The system is 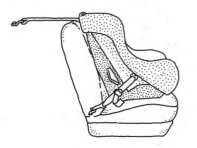 called Lower Anchors and Tethers for Children (LATCH), and it allows a car seat to be installed without using a vehicle's seat belt. With the LATCH system, two small bars, or anchors, are built right into the frame of the car; a lower anchor is at the base of the rear seat, and an upper anchor is usually at the top of the seat or in the vehicle's cargo area. A car seat attaches to each anchor with installation straps. New vehicles should have been equipped with the LATCH system by September 2002, and car safety seats should be sold with the necessary straps to use the system. If you are buying a new car or car seat, ask about the LATCH system.

When you buy a car seat, follow the recommendations of the American Academy of Pediatrics (AAP), which is online at www.aap.org.

AAP publishes a series of helpful guides, available on its website in the "parenting corner." Its guides include *Car Safety Seats: A Guide for Families, One-Minute Car Seat Safety Check-Up,* and *Safe Transportation of Children with Special Needs.* The 2005 AAP family guide for car seats includes the following recommendations:

- No one car seat is safest or best. When you find a seat you like, try it out with your child and in your vehicle. When the car seat is installed, be sure it does not move side to side or toward the front of the car. There are several types of car seat: infant-only, convertible, combination, booster, travel vest, and built-in. Each of these is described below.
- Infant-only seats can be used *only* in a rear-facing position. They are intended for infants up to one year old and up to about 20 pounds (varies with the model). These small, portable seats fit newborns best. Several models come with a convenient detachable base, so you can install the base in the vehicle and then just snap the car seat in and out of the base. If your child is younger than one year but weighs between 20 and 35 pounds, use a convertible seat instead. The child should still face the rear of the vehicle until she turns one year.

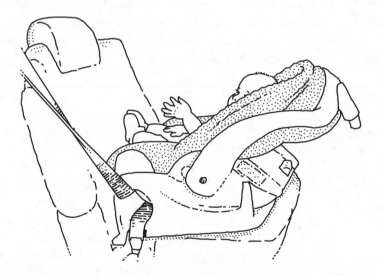

- Convertible seats can be used in both rear-facing and front-facing positions. They may not fit newborns as well as infant-only seats do, but they are just as safe for an infant and can be used for a longer time and for larger children. Use a convertible seat in its rear-facing position until an infant reaches at least one year of age *and* weighs at least 20 pounds. Follow the manufacturer's instructions for the proper recline angle. AAP recommends that as long as the top of the infant's head is below the top of the seat back, babies remain in rear-facing seats until they reach the maximum weight allowed by the model. A child who is at least one year old and weighs at least 20 pounds (but not more than 40 pounds) is ready to face forward in a car safety seat. When you switch a convertible seat to face forward, you need to make several adjustments (which will be described in the instruction booklet for the seat): move the shoulder straps to the slots above the child's shoulders; move the seat to the upright position; and route the vehicle's seat belt through the forward-facing belt path. Note that a convertible seat has two different belt paths, one for use in the rear-facing position and one for use forward-facing. Check the owner's manual for your car to find out if you need to use a locking clip, and check the car seat instructions to find out if you need a tether to keep the safety seat secure.

- Combination seats are only for children who are at least one year old and weigh at least 20 pounds. They cannot be used facing the rear. They convert to belt-positioning booster seats for children who weigh more than 40 pounds.

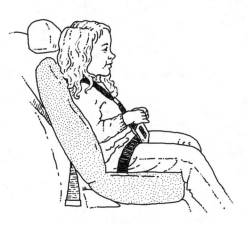

- Booster seats are for children who have reached the maximum weight allowed by a car seat, whose shoulders are above the harness slots, or whose ears have reached the top of the car seat. Use the booster seat until the child can correctly use the vehicle's seat belt, as described in the next point.
- A child is usually ready to use a vehicle's lap and shoulder belt when he reaches about 4'9" in height and 80 pounds and is between eight and twelve years old. When a vehicle's lap and shoulder belt are used correctly for a child, the shoulder belt lies across the middle of the chest, not across the neck or throat; the lap belt fits snugly across the thighs, not the stom-

ach; and the child sits against the back of the seat with his feet hanging down and his legs bent at the knee.

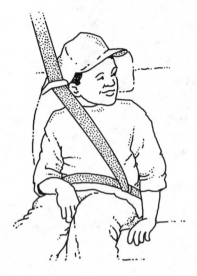

- Travel vests are an option if a vehicle has only lap belts. A travel vest is worn like a jacket and can be put on outside the vehicle. The shoulders of the vest attach to tethers that must be installed in the vehicle.
- Some vehicles have built-in child seats, which can be used for children who are at least one year old and weigh at least 20 pounds. Built-in seats eliminate installation problems, but weight and height limits vary. Check the vehicle manufacturer's instructions to be sure you use a built-in seat correctly.

Vehicle Travel Tips

1. Do not allow a child younger than twelve years to ride in the front seat. Airbags deploy at great speed and with great energy. They can kill a child passenger in the front seat.
2. Infants younger than one year old should ride in the back seat, facing the rear, and reclining at a 45-degree angle. This position protects the head, neck, and spinal cord from injury. Never carry a baby in your arms while riding in a vehicle.
3. Once a child reaches one year of age and weighs at least 20 pounds, the child should ride in the back seat, facing the front, and sitting upright.
4. When a child is at least three years old and weighs 30 to 60 pounds, she can use a booster seat. Use the seat's harness system until the child weighs about 40 pounds; then switch to using the vehicle's lap and shoulder belt with the booster seat.
5. Use a booster seat until a child is about eight years old or 80 pounds and can use the vehicle's lap and shoulder belt with a proper fit.

6. Read and follow the manufacturer's instructions. Pay particular attention to how the shoulder straps and their retaining clips need to be positioned. Keep instructions for future reference.

7. If the car seat has been involved in a vehicle crash, it may be damaged, even if it looks fine. It's best to buy a new car seat.

8. Beware of buying used car seats. You will likely have no way of knowing if the seat has been involved in a crash or if it meets current standards.

9. For airplane travel, the Federal Aviation Administration (FAA) and AAP recommend that children up to four years old be securely fastened in a child safety seat. Most infant, convertible, and forward-facing seats are certified for airplane use. Booster seats and travel vests are not. Check the label on the seat and call the airline before you travel to be sure the seat meets FAA regulations. Since August 2005 child safety seats are no longer mandated for airplane travel because the FAA found that if forced to purchase an extra airline ticket, families might choose to drive—a statistically more dangerous way to travel.

10. For answers to your questions and for a list of recalled car seats, call the Auto Safety Hotline (888-DASH-2-DOT or 888-327-4236), or check the National Highway Traffic Safety Administration (NHTSA) website (www.nhtsa.dot.gov).

11. Don't forget to buckle up yourself!

Key Actions to Prevent Vehicle Crash Injuries

To prevent or minimize injury to your child from motor vehicle incidents, do the following.

1. Always seat your child in a car seat or restraint system appropriate for her age and weight.

2. Be sure to install the seat correctly, according to its instructions.

3. Be sure to position the restraint correctly on your child's body, according to the seat's instructions.

4. Seat your child in the rear of the vehicle.

Got Wheels, Let's Go! Safety with Carriages and Strollers

With your child in a carriage or stroller, you can go just about any-where. And conveniently, you have a little extra storage space to stash items you need to take along and items you pick up or purchase on the way (but see below). Although carriages and strollers don't move nearly as quickly as motor vehicles (unless perhaps you push your child as you run a speed trial), they still present several hazards for infants and children. The most common injuries associated with strollers and carriages occur when a child falls out. Generally, a child falls out if he is not properly restrained or if he is able to disengage or wiggle out of the restraint. Carriages intended only for infants do not have a restraining system, but all other carriages and strollers must have one. You should always use the restraint, following the manufacturer's instructions for correct use.

Injuries associated with falling out of a carriage or stroller typically involve the face and head; most are treatable bruises and cuts, but fractures and internal injuries have been known to happen. One ten-month-old girl was left playing unrestrained in her stroller. Facing the back of the stroller, she stood up, lost her balance, and fell to the concrete floor. As she fell, her left foot was temporarily caught on the side of the stroller, so she landed on the left side of her head. Although she was hospitalized with a head injury, she recovered. Deaths are rare, but one or two occur each year and tend to be related to a child's becoming trapped (see below) rather than falling out. The risk of injury declines as a child gets older, because the child gains balance and so is less likely to fall out of a stroller; further, the child matures cognitively and is more apt to listen to your instructions, and she behaves more obediently and is more likely to remain restrained.

In the past, strollers and carriages were commonly involved in other serious injuries, such as fingertip amputation. There were also incidents of postural strangulation (strangling when the weight of a child's head or body presses him onto an object that blocks his airway). These kinds of injury have been greatly reduced because of a voluntary industry standard for carriages and strollers that covers stability, brakes, restraint systems, latches and folding mechanisms, structural integrity, and trapping. Strollers must now have a locking device that prevents unintentional folding. Make sure folding and latching mechanisms are in their correct position when you set up a stroller for use.

Strollers must also have leg openings too narrow to allow trapping

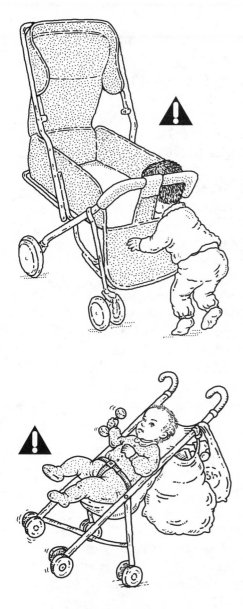

that could result in postural strangulation. Trapping incidents with the leg openings of strollers are less common now than in the past, but older strollers may still pose this hazard. Trapping sometimes occurred when an infant was napping in a stroller, out of a parent's direct view, while the footrest was in a lowered position. The child slipped both legs into one leg opening and fell partway through. The child's head, too large to pass through the opening, remained trapped, and the child strangled as a result of pressure on the neck. A four-month-old Texas boy was a victim of such a trapping injury. He was put to sleep for the night in a stroller, and when his mother checked on him about an hour later, she found him with his legs, arms, and trunk wedged through a leg opening, his head caught, and his feet resting on the floor. If you have an older stroller that might not meet the requirement to prevent trapping, then always raise the leg rest for a napping infant or child.

Finally, stroller tip-overs can occur when an adult uses a stroller to carry packages, usually on the handles or upper rear of the stroller. The excess weight causes instability, and the stroller tips, usually backward. This pattern is more likely with a younger child whose light weight cannot balance the added load. Strollers designed with storage space under the seat make a tip-over unlikely.

Key Actions to Prevent Stroller and Carriage Injuries

You can easily avoid injury to your child when using a stroller or carriage.

1. Always use the restraint system.
2. Fully engage any locks and latches.
3. Keep the leg rest raised for a sleeping infant or child.
4. If you carry packages on a stroller, place them in a way that keeps the stroller stable.

In You Get and Off We Go: Using Infant Carriers

Infants don't weigh a lot, so it's often easiest to carry them with you. Many parents and caregivers use infant carriers; some carriers are worn by the adult, while others are hand held. Bouncer seats are not really carriers, since they are usually used in a stationary position indoors, but for the sake of convenience I include them in the discussion below.

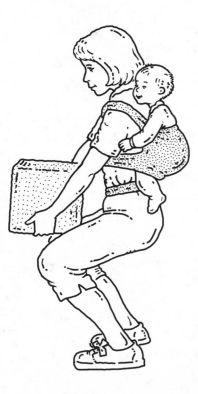

As with strollers and carriages, most injuries with carriers occur when an infant falls partly or completely out of the carrier or the carrier and the infant fall together. In carriers that are worn by an adult, falls can occur through the leg openings or from the top. When you wear a carrier, bend at your knees rather than at your waist. Falls from hand-held carriers have been caused by defective handles—if the handle gives way or disconnects, the baby can be tossed out—and by the whole carrier's falling off an elevated surface, such as a table or washing machine.

Falls from bouncer seats primarily occur from raised surfaces as well. Bouncer seats tend to move across a surface because of the baby's movements. Obviously, if a baby bounces her seat too close to the edge of a surface, she and the seat will fall off. Current voluntary standards for bouncer seats (2002) and hand-held carriers (2003) require that these products be made so they can't slip easily and so falls will be less likely. Remember that the floor is an excellent spot to rest a bouncer seat or a carrier.

Because young infants have poor muscle control, in carriers and

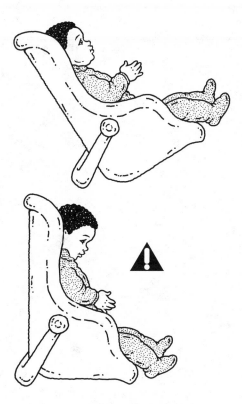

bouncer seats they are at risk of a particularly serious hazard: positional asphyxia (lack of oxygen). Infants can't yet fully support their head, so they should be positioned at about a 45-degree angle, not fully upright. If placed fully upright, they slump into a head-forward or head-down position that compromises breathing. Though nothing lies on or across the neck to strangle them, infants can still asphyxiate in scrunched-up positions. This scenario has occurred in both cloth sling carriers and hand-held carriers. Be sure to pay attention to the age recommendations for these products so that you don't use them for an infant who is too young or too old.

Carriers also pose suffocation hazards if they are placed on top of a bed, couch, or other soft surface. Parents may think that the surface will soften their child's fall should the carrier tip over. In reality the surface is unstable, encouraging the carrier to overturn; the baby is then trapped face down against the soft surface and can suffocate.

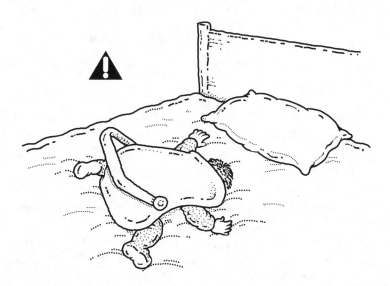

Another hazard with carriers involves a child's becoming tangled in the restraint straps and being strangled. An infant slips down in the carrier, and the straps get caught at the neck. Older infants may be attempting to get out of a carrier when this occurs. You can easily avoid this hazard by using a carrier that is age and weight appropriate and by fastening the restraints correctly.

⌇ Key Actions to Prevent Carrier Injuries

Reduce the chances of your infant or child's being injured in a carrier in the following ways.

1. Use a carrier that meets the age and weight requirements of your child.
2. Read all the instructions and warnings that come with the product.
3. Use the restraint, and be sure to position and adjust it according to the instructions.
4. Avoid placing a carrier on an elevated surface, but if you must, keep one hand on it and be well aware of the carrier's proximity to the edge.
5. Do not place your infant in her carrier on a bed, sofa, or other soft surface.

What's on the List? Safe Use of Shopping Carts

How many times have you seen children hanging on the outside of a shopping cart, standing in the basket, or sitting unrestrained in a cart's seat? Many times, probably. Shopping with a youngster can be a challenge, and trying to keep a child properly restrained adds to that challenge. But unrestrained children face a serious hazard: they can fall out of a shopping cart and be severely injured or even die. Between 1985 and 1994, the Consumer Product Safety Commission received three reports of children's death as a result of shopping-cart incidents. The children were aged six months, twelve months, and three years.

In more than half of shopping-cart injuries, children, especially boys, fall out of the cart. Little ones can fall from both the seat area and the basket area. Head, face, and mouth injuries are common, accounting for 63 percent of injuries when children fall from the basket and 94 percent of injuries when children fall from the seat. Concus-

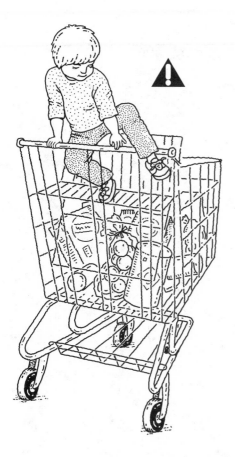

sions make up 20 percent of injuries from all shopping-cart falls. These statistics suggest that children are most likely to lose their balance and fall out of a shopping cart head first. To make matters worse, the flooring in grocery and department stores is typically linoleum, tile, or some other smooth, hard surface, probably laid down over cement. These surfaces don't absorb any energy from a fall, so a child's body takes the full force.

Two-year-old children are at highest risk of injury from shopping-cart falls: at this age children squirm, reach for items, and try to stand or climb out if the seat belt is either not available or not fastened. When falls occur, the adult accompanying the child tends to be close by, usually within six feet.

Injuries also result when a shopping cart's balance is upset and it tips over. Tip-overs can happen when a child climbs on the outside or leans out of a cart or when a cart rolls over uneven ground in a parking lot. Very young children can be injured when they are placed, in their infant carrier, into the basket of a shopping cart and the cart tips over. According to a report from the Department of Pediatric Surgery in an Austrian hospital, carts could be designed to better distribute weight and center of gravity to minimize tip-overs, but the U.S. voluntary industry standard (published in 2004) addresses only restraint systems and warning labels.

Key Actions to Prevent Shopping Cart Injuries

Keep your child safe with the following actions when you use a shopping cart.

1. Place your child who is six months to four years old and weighs at least 15 pounds, but not more than 35 pounds, into the seat and restrain her.

2. Do not allow your child to ride inside the basket.
3. Do not allow your child to hang on the outside of the basket.
4. When using a cart outdoors, avoid uneven terrain.
5. Instead of placing an infant carrier inside a shopping cart, consider using a stroller, backpack, or frontpack while shopping with a baby.

Summing Up

Travel is an everyday activity that includes potential for serious injury. In the United States, motor vehicle crashes will probably always be the leading cause of unintentional injury and death in children (and in adults too). Other less speedy types of transport—carriages, strollers, carriers, and shopping carts—are also associated with serious injury and death, though certainly on a much smaller scale. Proper restraint and placement of your child are key to minimizing injury, regardless of how you travel.

Travel Safely Checklist

Go through the following Travel Safely Checklist as you consider your child's travel environment.

1. Is your child always restrained when riding in a vehicle?
   Children should always be restrained when riding in a vehicle. Never hold a child in your lap.
2. Will your child ride in the vehicle's back seat until he reaches age twelve years?
   The safest place for all children to ride is in the back seat. Children older than twelve years may ride in the front seat.
3. Does your child sit in the correct car seat for her weight, height, and age?
   Follow the manufacturer's instructions for weight, height, and age to ensure that your child gets maximum protection from the seat.
4. When riding in a vehicle, is your child facing the correct way for his weight, height, and age?
   Infants should ride facing the back of the car until they have reached at least one year of age and weigh at least 20

pounds. A child who weighs more than 20 pounds and is older than one year may face forward.

5. Do you have the instructions for use of the car safety seat that your child rides in?

Follow the instructions and keep them, because you will need to refer to them again as your child grows. Be sure to send in the registration card that came with the car safety seat so the manufacturer knows to contact you if the seat is recalled.

6. Are the harness and straps positioned correctly on your child?

Follow the car seat manufacturer's instructions about how to adjust the straps.

7. Does your vehicle have the LATCH system for anchoring a car safety seat?

Lower Anchors and Tethers for Children (LATCH) is an anchor system that allows you to install a car safety seat without using the vehicle's seat belt. Most new vehicles and all new car safety seats have these attachments to secure the car seat in the vehicle. Unless both the vehicle and the car seat have this system, however, you still need to secure the car seat with the vehicle's seat belts.

8. Have you purchased a secondhand car seat for your child?

If you must use a secondhand car safety seat, first check its full history. Do not use a car safety seat that has been in a crash, has been recalled, has any cracks in its frame, is missing parts, or is too old (check with the manufacturer to find out if the seat complies with current safety standards). Make sure the seat has a label from the manufacturer and instructions. Call the car seat manufacturer if you have questions about the safety of the seat.

9. Has your child's car safety seat been recalled?

Call the Auto Safety Hotline (888-DASH-2-DOT or 888-327-4236) or check the National Highway Traffic Safety Administration (NHTSA) website (www.nhtsa.dot.gov) for a list of recalled seats. Be sure to make any needed repairs, per the manufacturer's recall instructions, to your car safety seat.

10. Has your child's car safety seat ever been in a crash?

If the seat has been in a crash, it may have been weakened and should not be used, even if it does not look damaged.

11. Once your child of about four years outgrows her car safety seat, do you use a belt-positioning booster seat to help pro-

tect her until she is big enough for the vehicle's seat belt to fit properly?

A booster seat helps to keep a child safe during the transition time between use of a car seat and use of a vehicle's seat belt. A belt-positioning booster seat is used with the vehicle's lap and shoulder belt.

12. Once your child begins using a booster seat, and after he graduates from a booster seat, do you know how a vehicle's seat belt should fit?

A seat belt fits properly when the shoulder belt crosses the chest and the lap belt is low and snug across the thighs. A child should use the vehicle's seat belt only when he is tall enough for his legs to bend at the knee and for his feet to hang down while he sits against the back of the vehicle's seat.

13. When using a soft carrier, do you follow the age and weight recommendations?

Follow the product's instructions to minimize the risk of your child's falling through a leg opening or over the top. Face the child according to the product instructions.

14. When your child rides in a carriage or stroller, do you use the restraint?

Always use the restraint and fasten it correctly to prevent your child from falling out of the carriage or stroller.

15. If your baby falls asleep in a stroller, do you raise the leg rest?

Some strollers may have large leg openings that can allow a child to slip through feet first. The head is too large to pass through the leg opening, so the slipped child can strangle because of her body position. While you are out with the stroller, be sure to raise the leg rest for your sleeping child; when you get home, transfer your sleeping baby to her crib.

16. When your child of age six months to four years (maximum 35 pounds) rides in a shopping cart, do you use the restraint?

Always use the restraint and fasten it correctly to prevent your child from falling out of the shopping cart.

17. Do you allow older siblings to ride inside the shopping cart or to hang onto the outside?

Do not allow children to ride inside or outside a shopping cart. Children inside the basket can stand and fall out; children on the outside can upset the cart's balance and cause it to tip over.

7

Upstairs, Downstairs, and All Around the House

Young children spend most of their time at home, even if they go to daycare. Apartments and houses tend to be designed for adults, however, and so young children live primarily in an adult world, whether it's the kitchen, bathroom, living room, laundry room, backyard, or another area. A child's bedroom or nursery is easiest to keep safe, because it most likely contains items made for children, according to safety standards. But parents and caregivers need to be aware of how to alter other home spaces to make them safer for children. Sometimes the solution is as simple as keeping a child out of a particular room by using a baby gate or restricting a child's movement in a room by using a playpen. Other times you may need to install safety items, such as child locks on cabinets and toilet lids. Obviously, your child's age, mobility, and curiosity will all affect how much you will need to change the general household environment.

This chapter discusses potential hazards and injury situations typically found in a home, including the backyard. In the next chapter, I walk you through a home, room by room, to point out specific hazards. It would be impossible to cover all conceivable hazards, since there is tremendous variation among individual homes and the ways individuals use rooms and spaces in their homes. So this chapter and the next chapter will highlight particularly serious hazards that are addressed in the professional literature but may not be well recognized as hazards by parents and caregivers.

A Breath of Fresh Air: Indoor Air Quality

The quality of the air you breathe inside your home plays a significant role in your overall health. Allergies, headaches, skin irritations, asthma, and other health problems can arise because of chemicals or organisms in indoor air. Often, indoor air pollutants are invisible and odorless, so it is hard to detect a problem. For example, carbon monoxide, a natural and odorless byproduct of burning fuel, can contaminate indoor air and cause fatigue, headache, nausea, and even death. Because of the serious consequences of breathing air laden with carbon monoxide, there are several things to remember about burning fuel:

- Fuel-driven (as opposed to electrically operated) appliances, such as furnaces, space heaters, gas clothes dryers, gas fireplaces, wood-burning stoves, hot water tanks, and other similar products, must be vented to the outdoors.
- Never burn charcoal indoors.
- Never start a car in a garage when the garage door is closed.

Another source of carbon monoxide is smoking. A lit cigarette, pipe, or cigar produces smoke, and the smoker exhales smoke. Together, these two sources are known as *secondhand smoke*. Besides carbon monoxide, secondhand smoke contains numerous other harmful chemicals, many identified as carcinogens—cancer-causing chemicals. Secondhand smoke is a health hazard for everyone, but it is particularly dangerous for infants and young children, because their organ systems are developing. Infants exposed to secondhand smoke have far higher levels of smoke-related toxins in their saliva and urine than do the adult smokers who expose them to smoke. Children exposed to secondhand smoke are more likely to have respiratory illnesses, like bronchitis and pneumonia, than children not exposed to it. They are also more likely to have asthma. Even if a smoker blows smoke away from other people, smokes in a different room, or opens a window, children will still be exposed to secondhand smoke. If you or a family member smokes, try to quit or encourage the other person to quit, and seek help from a doctor if necessary. If this doesn't work, smoke outdoors, and insist that visitors smoke outdoors, too.

There is one additional concern regarding tobacco smoke. The combination of tobacco smoke and radon—a colorless, odorless gas formed by the natural decay of uranium—increases the risk of lung cancer. Uranium is found in soil and rocks and is more prevalent in certain parts of the United States, like the West. Basements, which tend not to be well ventilated, are more likely to have elevated levels of radon than other parts of the home. If you wish to test for radon in your home, you can buy a test kit at a hardware store.

Another aspect of indoor air is dust—the ubiquitous mix of soil tracked in from outdoors, chemicals from outdoor air, residues of chemical products used indoors, animal and human dander, insects and their droppings, and mildew and mold. Although the makeup of dust varies with the time of year, household habits, and geographic location, dust is a constant problem. A runny nose, runny and itchy eyes, and itchy skin can be related to house dust. Dust mites—bugs so small that we can't see them—live in bedding, pillows, and carpets. These nasty little creatures excrete a liquid that can cause an allergic reaction in people.

Indoor air quality can also be affected by some of the actions we take to counter a different problem. For example, you may be able to solve an insect problem by using pesticides, but spraying a pesticide indoors contributes to pollution. Even products used on animals, like flea and tick powders and collars, dips, and shampoos, can increase the possibility of allergic reactions. Children are often most affected by animal products, because children tend to hug pets and stay closer to them than adults do.

❧ Key Actions to Maintain the Quality of Indoor Air

You can do several basic things around your home to keep the indoor air quality as good as possible.

1. Regularly change air filters on the furnace and air ducts.
2. Make sure that woodstoves, fireplaces, and fuel-driven space heaters and appliances are vented to the outside, and have them inspected annually.
3. Install carbon monoxide detectors—they are relatively inexpensive and easy to install, and they operate just like smoke detectors. As of March 31, 2006, the state of Massachusetts required carbon monoxide detectors to be installed in residences that have fuel-burning (oil, gas, wood, coal) equipment or that have enclosed parking, such as an attached garage. Some other U.S. states have passed similar laws. Remember to change your detector's batteries regularly. (An

easy rule of thumb is to change the batteries in carbon mon-oxide and smoke detectors each time you change the clocks between standard and daylight savings time.)

4. Do not allow people to smoke indoors.
5. Before entering the house, wipe your feet on a doormat to minimize outdoor soil and pollutants on the soles of your shoes.
6. For any chemical product you use indoors, follow the use and ventilation instructions.
7. Dust, vacuum, and mop regularly.
8. Use hypoallergenic bedding for sensitive children.

Up, Down, Open, Shut: Staying Safe around Stairs and Windows

Once your infant is mobile, you must think about where he might go and how he might get there. Stairs, in particular, become a hazard for falls. Many infants—especially those seated in walkers—have ended up at the bottom of a flight of stairs. Walkers are used less often than in the past; today, stationary entertainment centers are more common. It's best not to use an infant walker, but if you do, be sure to use a walker that meets the latest safety standard (2003 as of this book's publication). The standard requires walkers to be larger than a standard doorway or to be equipped with a gripping mechanism that prevents them from toppling over an edge.

Baby gates are effective at denying a child's access to stairs. Install

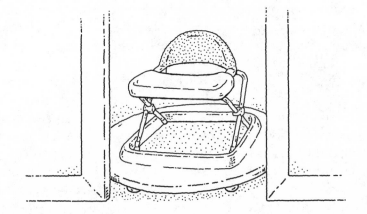

gates at both the top and the bottom of stairs. Gates bear a label indicating whether they are appropriate for use at the top of stairs. Those approved for use at the top have a more stringent safety requirement than those for use at the bottom. Be sure to use only a gate intended for the top of stairs at that location. In addition, use only gates made after 1985, because earlier gates were a trapping hazard.

Windows attract children, as they do adults, but for children they pose two hazards: a child can fall out of an open window, and a child can be injured by blinds and other types of window covering.

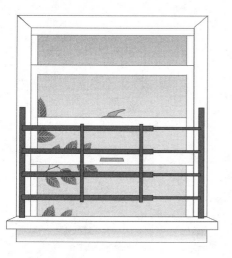

For a child, the interest in being able to see out a window makes her want to lean out, and if she leans too far, she may fall out. Children five years and younger who live in apartment buildings are at the greatest risk of falling out of windows. You can easily prevent such a fall, however, by using fall prevention devices. Also known as window guards, these devices are specially designed with horizontal bars to prevent a child from fitting through a window. The window can still open all the way when a window guard is in place. Note that insect screens are *not* window guards and do not prevent children from falling out of windows. Window guards also differ from security or burglar bars, which are intended to keep someone from getting in and are usually installed at ground level. Some security bars can double as window guards, though, if their design meets the window guard standard.

Some cities and locales require window guards in certain buildings. For example, since 1976 the New York City Board of Health has mandated that protective window guards be installed on all windows (except emergency exits) in multifamily buildings where children younger than ten years live. In 1993, Boston developed a Kids Can't Fly program, which included public education and voluntary installation of window guards. Other communities across the United States have similar requirements or programs in place. These efforts have dramatically reduced the incidence of childhood falls from windows.

Any window coverings that have a looped cord—blinds, in particular—pose a strangling or hanging hazard. Any cord or string with a loop large enough to fit over a child's head can become a noose. Children can hang in a standing, sitting, kneeling, or lying position; they do not have to have their feet off the ground to hang. So for all accessible windows, no matter how close to the floor, ensure that there are no looped cords or any other feature that could create a loop.

When you arrange the furniture in your child's bedroom, place the crib or bed well away from windows. Children can stand in a crib, reach out, and pull a blind or shade cord into their crib (see illustration on p. 31). Children also tend to play on beds and can unintentionally jump out a window or be pushed out a window. Similarly, do not place dressers, tables, and other furniture under or beside windows, because children can climb on furniture and gain access to both the window and the window covering.

❦ Key Actions to Prevent Staircase and Window Injuries

You can keep your child safe around stairs and windows throughout your home.

1. Use secure baby gates at the top and bottom of stairs.
2. Have your infant play in a stationary entertainment center instead of putting him in a walker.
3. If you live in a multifamily high-rise, install window guards on all windows in your home. If you live in a house, consider installing window guards for windows on the second floor and higher.
4. Remove all loops from window cords that dangle; cut the loop and retie the ends separately.
5. Place furniture far enough from windows that your child cannot climb up and access the window or the window covering.

Sweet but Deadly: What Are the Hazards of Lead?

People have used lead for centuries—in fact, the Romans had lead pipes for their water supply and sweetened their wine with lead. In recent times, products such as gasoline and paint contained lead additives. But now we know that lead, an element found naturally on Earth, can poison people, affecting their behavior and development. Lead is particularly dangerous for children because it causes brain and nervous system damage, including lower IQ. Lead poisoning has also been associated with hyperactivity, withdrawal from social interaction, anemia, blindness, and damage to other organs, such as bones and kidneys. Children who are exposed to lead absorb more of the element into their bodies than adults do.

Much has been done to reduce the amount of lead in our environment. For example, lead is no longer present in gasoline, and leaded paint has been banned since 1978. However, some older homes still have leaded paint, which puts children at high risk of lead poisoning. Children eat paint chips and ingest lead dust from their fingers and toys when they play on the floor. Lead can also be inhaled as dust in the air.

Lead solder used to be used in plumbing, so older plumbing can affect the lead content of drinking water. Water that has been sitting unused in an older pipe for a long time, such as overnight, has the highest lead content. If you suspect the pipes in your home are old, let the water run a bit before using it at the start of the day, and always start with cold water when you cook.

As recently as 1996, the Consumer Product Safety Commission found that imported vinyl miniblinds contained lead. The vinyl deteriorates in the sun and in heat, producing lead dust. When you buy miniblinds, look for a label that specifies "non-leaded formula" or "no lead added." In spite of regulations against the use of lead, it is still possible that some imported products, such as glazed pottery, may contain it. If you have items that contain lead or if you are unsure, do not use them as food containers, because the lead can leach into the food, especially acidic food like fruit juice.

Key Actions to Prevent Lead Poisoning

Keep your child safe from the behavioral and developmental problems associated with lead.

1. If your home was built before 1978, have the paint checked, and if it contains lead, have it removed by professionals.
2. If your water pipes are old, let water run about two minutes before using it in the morning. Start with cold water when you cook.
3. Check vinyl miniblinds for labels stating that they are lead free.
4. If you are concerned that your child may have been exposed to lead, ask your doctor about lead testing.
5. Have children wash their hands before eating or snacking.

Fire Prevention and Safety

Fire can break out in any room and spread quickly throughout an entire house. Most fire-related deaths are caused by inhalation of the toxic fumes created during a fire, while about one quarter of fire-related deaths result from severe burns. You can minimize the risk of fire and the consequences of fire if you recognize and avoid fire hazards, equip your home with smoke detectors, and practice fire drills with your children.

By age twelve, nearly half of all children have played with fire. Boys are about twice as likely as girls to play with fire. Children's "play fires" are the leading cause of residential fire-related deaths and injuries among children aged nine years and younger. Children as young as three years have used multipurpose lighters (the long-handled lighters convenient for lighting barbecues and fireplaces) to inadvertently start house fires, while older children have used cigarette lighters and matches. For good reason, cigarette lighters, novelty lighters, and multipurpose lighters are required by federal law to be child resistant. Remember, though, that children younger than five years may still be able to operate a child-resistant product. "Child resistance" does not guarantee that young children will find a product impossible to use. So keep lighters, matches, and similar products out of children's reach, and teach older children about the dangers of open flames.

Household fires can also start in numerous other ways, some of which are not obvious. How many of the following examples are new to you?

- When used or stored in dangerous ways, flammable substances such as mineral spirits and gasoline can ignite and cause fires. Not only the liquid can catch fire; the vapors from flammable products can also catch fire or even explode. This is a particularly insidious hazard, because vapors are usually invisible. Flammable substances must be labeled by law, so they are easy to identify, provided they are left in their original container. If you use or store flammable substances indoors, do so well away from ignition sources, which include open flames, sparks, pilot lights, heaters, and smoking materials. Also ensure adequate ventilation when using flammable substances indoors so that vapors do not accumulate. When you have finished using a flammable product, make sure to cap it tightly.

Store flammables in their original containers. Ideally, you will store fuel-run equipment (like a gas lawn mower) in a garage or shed. If you must store lawn mowers and other fuel-run equipment inside, run them until they are completely out of fuel before storage, and never store them near an ignition or heat source.

- Pilot lights are open flames on gas furnaces, hot water heaters, and fireplaces. When lighting a pilot light, follow directions carefully, and allow adequate time for the gas to dissipate after unsuccessful attempts at lighting. Accumulated gas can explode when you light the next match or lighter.

- Kerosene heaters can reach a surface temperature of 700° F or hotter, so nearby flammable materials can ignite. Place a kerosene heater at least three feet away from anything that can burn, including draperies, bedding, and clothing. Turn the heater off at night and when you leave the house. It is also a good idea to check with local authorities about using a kerosene heater, because some locales restrict or ban their use in certain kinds of homes.

- Electricity can start a house fire, often when electrical cords or circuits are overloaded or damaged. Check electrical cords regularly, and discard or get repaired any that are frayed or otherwise damaged. Use extension cords only when absolutely necessary, and run them along the wall rather than under carpets where they will be walked on. If you do use an extension cord, be sure that it is graded for the use you have in mind. It is also a good idea to unplug small electrical appliances, like toasters, when they are not in use.

- Electric space heaters have started fires when used to thaw frozen water pipes. In these cases, the heat generated by the heater ignited nearby flammable materials, like insulation. If you use an electric space heater, place it at least three feet away from anything that can burn, and be sure to turn it off at night and when you leave the house.

- Candles have become quite popular and are often involved in house fires. Read the directions that accompany candles and candle holders. Burn candles only within your view, and place them well away from anything that could ignite. When you leave the house, leave a room, or go to sleep, be sure to extinguish candles.

- Kitchen fires during cooking, whether the stove is gas or electric, are also common. Hot grease forgotten on a stove, or transferred to another container to cool, or a pan whose contents have boiled away can catch fire and ignite nearby flammables. Stay at the stove when you are cooking, and let hot grease cool in the cooking pan rather than transferring it to another container.

- Warm fireplace ashes have burned through bags in which they were placed and have set fire to entire homes. Make sure ashes are cool to the touch before bagging and discarding them.
- Falling asleep while smoking has been a classic cause of house fires. If you smoke, do so sitting up, not reclining, and never in bed.

As well as eliminating fire hazards from your home, you would be wise—and in some places you are legally obligated—to install smoke detectors. Smoke detectors should be installed on each floor, especially near bedrooms. A smoke detector will be of use only if it functions properly, so make sure to replace the batteries at least once a year or when you hear the detector chirping. As mentioned earlier, a helpful reminder is to change the batteries every time you change the clock between standard time and daylight savings time so that you will always have functioning batteries. Be aware that detectors wired directly into a house's electricity may also have a battery backup, and these batteries should be changed as frequently as those in battery-operated detectors.

Installing and maintaining smoke detectors can save your life and the lives of your children. Resist the urge to disable a detector to stop annoying false alarms. A disabled smoke detector denies you its critical role when you really need it. If a detector goes off in nuisance fashion—for example, in response to cooking—try changing its location. According to the Safe Kids organization, in two of every three residential fires in which a child is injured or killed, a working smoke detector is lacking. In addition, households without working detectors are two and a half times more likely to have a fire than those with working detectors. The chances of dying in a fire are halved by the presence of a smoke detector.

Create an escape plan in case your home catches on fire. Children tend to panic and hide when fire breaks out, so that rescue becomes difficult. To reduce their panic, regularly practice the escape plan with your children. If they are used to carrying out the plan, children are more likely to follow it and escape a fire. As part of your escape plan,

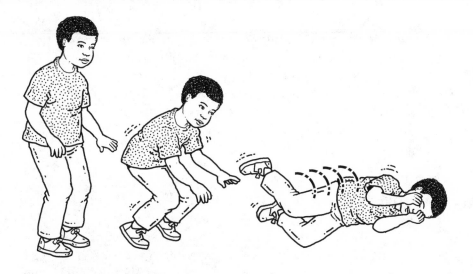

designate a meeting place outside your home. Also teach children that if their clothing catches on fire, they should "stop, drop, and roll" to put the flames out quickly.

ᛋ Key Actions to Prevent Fire and Be Prepared for Fire

There are several ways you can minimize the risk of fire in your home. In the event that fire does break out, your prior preparation will increase your and your family's chances of escaping the blaze.

1. Store matches and lighters, including child-resistant lighters, in a location that your child can't reach.
2. Store flammable substances and fuel-driven equipment in a shed or garage rather than a basement. If flammable substances must be stored inside, keep their containers tightly capped and away from ignition sources. If equipment must be stored inside, run it dry and store it away from ignition sources.
3. Light pilot lights according to product instructions, and allow gas to dissipate after an unsuccessful attempt at lighting a pilot light.
4. Keep kerosene heaters, space heaters, and candles at least three feet away from materials that could ignite. Turn heaters off if you leave the house or go to sleep, and extinguish candles if you leave the room or go to sleep.

5. Run extension cords along the wall, and check all electrical cords for damage, fixing or replacing them if necessary.
6. Install smoke detectors on each floor of your home, and change the batteries regularly.
7. Create a fire escape plan, including a designated meeting place, and practice the plan regularly with your family.
8. Teach your child to stop, drop, and roll if her clothing catches on fire.

Firearms: Preventing Gun-Related Tragedies

In 2004, according to the National Safe Kids Campaign, Americans owned nearly 200 million firearms, including 65 million handguns. Guns kept in the home for protection were usually handguns, they were most often found in a home with children, and they tended to be stored loaded and unlocked. Approximately one-third of families with children had at least one gun in their home.

A gun in the home is extremely dangerous for children. Parents and caregivers commonly *under*estimate a child's ability to find a gun and to fire one, while they *over*estimate children's ability to distinguish between toy and real guns and to follow rules about gun safety. Children as young as three years are strong enough to pull the trigger of many of the handguns available in the United States. Before age eight, few children can reliably distinguish between toy and real guns, and children cannot fully understand the consequences of their actions.

In one devastating incident, two Texas brothers, aged two and four years, were fighting over a toy. The older boy went to his mother's purse and got her handgun—the only time it hadn't been locked up, she claimed—and shot his brother in the temple. The four-year-old did not understand what he had done, and he kept asking where his brother was and when he was coming back.

Unintentional shootings among children occur most often when children are unsupervised and out of school. These shootings tend to happen in the late afternoon (peaking between 4:00 and 5:00 p.m.), on weekends, in the summer months (June to August), and over the holiday season (November to December). Boys are much more likely than girls to be involved in unintentional shootings.

To prevent firearm-related injury and death among children, it is imperative that firearms be stored safely, in ways that eliminate their availability and accessibility to children. Every incident in which a child aged five years or younger shot and killed himself or another person could have been prevented by a safety device, such as a gun lock. At least eighteen states have enacted child access prevention (CAP) laws, which may hold adults criminally liable for failing to store loaded firearms in a place inaccessible to children and for failing to use safety devices to lock a gun.

✦ Key Actions to Prevent Firearm-Related Injury and Death

You should seriously consider the risks of keeping a gun in your home. If you choose to keep a firearm—including a BB or pellet gun—keep children safe in the following ways.

1. Store your firearm unloaded and locked up, out of reach of children.
2. Lock ammunition in a separate location, also out of reach of children.
3. Use quality safety devices, like gun locks, lock boxes, and gun safes, with every gun kept in the home.
4. Keep gun storage keys and lock combinations hidden in a separate location.

In the Backyard: Safety Outdoors

Children love to play outside, and their home's backyard is often the area where they spend much of their outdoor time. While they are outside playing games and running about, they can encounter a number of hazards. Common backyard hazards include motorized equipment, gardening products, and even some plants. Hazards from water in the backyard are described in the section following this one.

When you are mowing the lawn or trimming greenery, have your children stay indoors. Cutters and trimmers can kick back and throw rocks and other debris. As the user of such equipment, keep yourself safe by wearing eye protection and appropriate clothing and footwear, and keep bystanders safe by insisting that they stay at least twenty feet away. It's safest for children to remain indoors until you finish using the equipment. Ride-on lawn mowers pose a particularly high risk of injury to children. In some cases, children have been run over by a ride-on lawn mower because the operator was backing up and couldn't see the child. In other cases, children have been injured

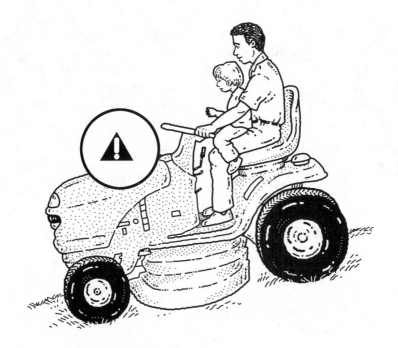

when riding on a mower that tipped over on a hill or grade. Never allow a child to ride with you on a mower.

Many homeowners use gardening products such as fertilizers, weed
and insect killers, and other lawn and garden chemicals. All of these
garden products can be extremely poisonous, so keep them in a locked
shed. Some products should not be applied if children or animals are
likely to be in the area—or children and animals should be kept out
of the area for a certain number of days following application. Be sure
to read product instructions.

Bushes and shrubbery, lovely though they are for shade and pri-
vacy, can be breeding grounds for ticks and disease-carrying rodents.
Keep bushes and other plants well trimmed to minimize these problems. Many plants are poisonous—it is surprising how many plants
contain toxins in their berries, flowers, or leaves. Check with your local poison control center to find out if any of the plants in your yard
are poisonous, and either remove them or install fencing or some
other barrier around them.

You may also consider installing a fence or planting shrubs around
part of your backyard to create a safe outdoor environment for your
child away from street traffic. Explain to your children the danger of
dashing out onto the street after a toy that's gone astray.

⟨ Key Actions for Backyard Safety

The backyard is a great place for your child to play, provided you keep a few hazards in mind and take actions to prevent injury.

1. Keep children indoors while the lawn is being mowed. Never let your child ride on a mower with you.
2. Store gardening chemicals in a locked area inaccessible to your child.
3. Keep bushes trimmed, and find out whether you have poisonous plants in your yard.
4. Consider installing a fence or planting shrubs around your backyard.

Water, Water, Everywhere: How to Prevent Pool, Bucket, and Other Backyard Drowning

Children are attracted to water, wherever it happens to be. They love to scamper through puddles, splash in pools, and slosh water about in buckets and other containers. Most parents want their children to be comfortable in and around water and to learn how to swim at a young age. But familiarity with water is one thing and safety another. No matter how comfortable your young child seems to be in and around water, remember that she is not aware of the possibility of drowning. According to a May 2002 press release from the Consumer Product Safety Commission, about 350 children younger than five years drown in home swimming pools each year. Other, perhaps less recognized, drowning sites include spas, hot tubs, ponds, and buckets, especially reused five-gallon buckets (used to hold liquids while washing a car or floor, for example).

Above-ground pools don't necessarily need to be fenced, provided that steps and ladders to the pool are secured and locked or removed when the pool is not in use. But backyard in-ground pools should have fences (or other barriers) that are at least four feet high and that extend around all four sides of the pool, or around three sides if the house forms the fourth side. Fences that can be climbed—for example, chain link fences—are not suitable around pools. Fence gates should open outward from the pool and be self-closing and self-latching, with the latch higher than a child's reach. Regardless of the kind of pool you have, check with local authorities to ensure that you follow any regulations about pool fencing.

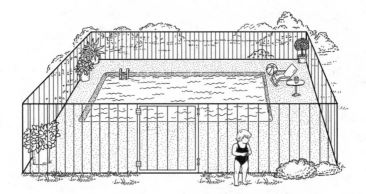

If the house forms one side of the pool barrier, doors leading from the house to the pool should be equipped with an alarm system. You may also consider installing a pool alarm, which responds to water motion when a child (or an object) falls into the pool. A safety cover provides a barrier over the water and can be used when the pool is not in use. Be careful not to let water collect on top of the cover, though, because children have drowned in pool-cover puddles.

When your pool is in use—whether it is an above-ground or in-ground pool—keep a telephone and emergency numbers poolside. Also keep basic lifesaving equipment, such as a pole, rope, and flotation device, nearby. When the pool is not in use, put away floats, toys, and other pool items that might attract a child.

If a child is missing, look in the pool first. Brain damage and drowning happen very quickly. A child goes unconscious only two minutes after being submersed in water, and irreversible brain damage occurs after four to six minutes of submersion. Most children who drown are found after ten minutes in the water. Learn CPR so that you have the best possible chance of saving a child who falls into a pool or other water source.

Pools account for many backyard drownings but not for all of them. Children have also drowned in hot tubs and spas. About half of all children younger than five years who drown in hot tubs and spas are in the twelve- to twenty-three-month age range. When older children drown in hot tubs and spas, the drowning tends to occur because their hair or a body part becomes trapped in suction fittings while they play underwater. Secure a backyard hot tub or spa as you would a swimming pool, so that young children do not have access to it. Children younger than twelve should not be allowed in hot tubs and spas, even if an adult is present.

Backyard ponds and creeks also present a drowning hazard. These bodies of water are difficult to enclose. In addition, they are often valued for the beauty they add to a backyard, so you wouldn't want to encircle them with fencing or other visual obstructions. If you have children younger than three years, it is best to avoid a yard with a pond or creek.

Another backyard drowning hazard that you might not think of is a septic tank. If you have a septic tank at ground level, padlock the lid. A two-year-old boy who had been missing for about a half-hour was found drowned in the septic tank of his backyard. Apparently the cover of the tank had not been secured.

Consumer Product Safety Alert

FROM THE U.S. CONSUMER PRODUCT SAFETY COMMISSION, WASHINGTON, D.C. 20207

Infants & Toddlers Can Drown in 5-Gallon Buckets

A Hidden Hazard In The Home

Large buckets and young children can be a deadly combination. The U.S. Consumer Product Safety Commission (CPSC) has received reports of over 275 young children who have drowned in buckets since 1984. Over 30 other children have been hospitalized. Almost all of the containers were 5-gallon buckets containing liquids. Most were used for mopping floors or other household chores. Many were less than half full.

Of all buckets, the 5-gallon size presents the greatest hazard to young children because of its tall, straight sides and weight, even with just a small amount of liquid. At 14-inches high, a 5-gallon bucket is about half the height of a young child. That, combined with the stability, makes it nearly impossible for top-heavy infants and toddlers to free themselves when they fall into the bucket head first. A child can drown in a small amount of water.

Children are naturally curious and easily attracted to water. At the crawling and pulling up stages while learning to walk, they can quickly get into trouble. CPSC believes that bucket drownings happen when children are left momentarily unattended, crawl to a bucket, pull themselves up, and lean forward to reach for an object or play in the water.

Parents and caregivers who are using 5-gallon buckets for household chores are warned not to leave a bucket containing even a small amount of liquid unattended where a young child may gain access to it. A child can drown in the time it takes to answer a telephone.

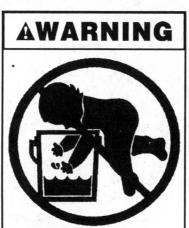

⚠WARNING

Children can fall into bucket and drown.

Keep children away from bucket with even a small amount of liquid.

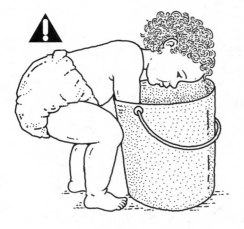

In the four-year period from 1996 to 1999, fifty-eight children younger than five years drowned in reused five-gallon buckets. The drownings occurred in spite of a standard requiring these products to carry a warning label. Five-gallon buckets are so hazardous because their tall, straight sides make them quite stable. When a child falls into a bucket, the bucket remains upright, and it is nearly impossible for the child to get out. Toddlers are at greatest risk of bucket drownings, because a toddler's high center of gravity makes him fall over easily once he begins to bend. If you use five-gallon buckets, look to see if they have a warning label—had you noticed the label before? (The Safety Alert from the Consumer Product Safety Commission is reproduced in its entirety on page 139 to provide an example of the label and of how the Commission informs the public of this kind of hazard.) When you use these buckets, get into the habit of emptying them immediately after use and storing them out of children's reach. Left uncovered outside, the buckets can collect rainwater and pose a drowning risk. Remember that a child can drown in even a few inches of liquid.

⤙ Key Actions to Prevent Backyard Drownings

You can take several precautions to keep your child safe around water and to be prepared in the event that an incident happens.

1. Install four-foot fences around in-ground pools, and lock or remove stairs from above-ground pools.
2. Keep lifesaving equipment, emergency phone numbers, and a telephone next to the pool.
3. Stay with your child whenever she plays in or around water.
4. Empty buckets immediately after you finish your chore. Store buckets out of children's reach and where the buckets won't fill with rainwater.
5. Padlock the lid of a ground-level septic tank.
6. Learn CPR, and take a refresher course regularly.

Summing Up

Infants and young children spend most of their time at home, yet homes tend to be designed and built for adults more than for children. Some hazards around the home—lead in particular—are a major concern only in older houses, but most of the hazards discussed in this chapter could occur in any home. As a parent or caregiver, you can eliminate or minimize common health and injury hazards associated with your home, both indoors and out.

Household Environment Safety Checklist

Consider your home environment in light of the following Household Environment Safety Checklist.

Indoor Air Quality
1. Does anyone in your household smoke?

    Smoking is the source of many dangerous chemicals. The hazards of these chemicals affect infants and children more than they do adults. Protect your child from secondhand smoke by asking smokers to smoke outside, not inside.
2. Do you know the common sources of indoor carbon monoxide?

    Carbon monoxide is a colorless, odorless toxic gas that can cause fatigue, headaches, and even death if enough of it accumulates in the body. Besides secondhand smoke, other common sources of carbon monoxide are faulty venting of fuel-burning appliances, like gas furnaces and kerosene heaters, faulty venting of wood-burning stoves and fireplaces, and car exhaust.
3. Do you know how to monitor carbon monoxide levels in your home?

    You can buy a carbon monoxide detector to monitor household levels of the gas. If the level of carbon monoxide is too high, you will need to do some detective work to figure out the source and get it repaired.
4. Do you or your children have itchy eyes, a runny nose, asthma, wheezing, or other respiratory symptoms?

    If so, you may have a problem with dust or another pollutant. Some good ways to control indoor pollutants include changing heater and air-conditioner filters regularly, opening windows so fresh air can circulate indoors, minimizing the use of pesticides indoors unless you can properly ventilate or leave for the time it takes for fumes to dissipate, and mopping and dusting regularly.

Stairs and Windows

1. If you have an infant or toddler, do you use baby gates at the top and bottom of stairs?

   Falls down stairs are common. A gate makes an effective barrier to keep youngsters from tumbling down stairs. At the top of a flight of stairs, be sure to use a gate that is specifically designed for that location.

2. Does your infant use a walker?

   Walkers are no longer recommended, because they give children greater speed and greater access to hazards. The most common type of injury with infant walkers was a fall down a set of stairs. Stationary play centers have become popular and are preferable to mobile walkers.

3. Do any of the blinds or window decorations in your home have loops?

   Children, especially those younger than three years old, are at high risk for hanging in cords that form loops. If you find loops, cut them and retie them as two individual cords.

4. Are cribs and beds placed away from windows?

   Keeping cribs and beds away from windows removes the hazard of hanging or becoming tangled in window decorations and helps prevent falls from windows.

5. If you live in a high-rise building or a house with upper floors, are the windows equipped with window guards?

   Remember that insect screens do not prevent children from falling out a window; only window guards do. Falls from windows, especially those above the second floor, can result in serious injury or death.

Lead

1. Do you live in a house built before 1978?

   If you do, have you had it checked for lead-containing paint? Today's paints must meet a federal requirement that bans the use of lead.

2. Do you know why lead is such a problem for young children?

   Lead is a toxin that attacks the nervous system and brain, causing lowered IQ, myriad illnesses, and social and behavioral dysfunctions. Young children's bodies absorb more lead than adults' bodies do.

3. Does your home have lead pipes?

   Lead in drinking water is associated with lead plumbing. Lead from the pipes leaches into the water. If you have lead pipes and have not run the water for a while, let it run for two minutes before using any water, and always cook starting with cold water.

Fire

1. Where do you store matches and lighters?

   Lighters have to be child resistant, but that does not mean that a child younger than five years will never be able to operate one. Many children play with fire and start house fires. Thus you must store matches and lighters out of your child's reach. Remember that children climb, so choose a storage spot with that in mind.

2. Where and how do you store flammables like gasoline, turpentine, and glue?

   Substances like these, and their vapors, are flammable, so you must store them tightly capped and away from ignition sources. Ignition sources include pilot lights on gas furnaces and heaters, open flames, sparks, and lit cigarettes.

3. Do you keep lit candles in view at all times and away from flammables?

   Unattended candles are a common cause of house fires. When you light candles, set them a good distance from draperies, clothing, and other materials that could catch fire. When you leave a room, put the candle out. Do not leave candles burning in rooms where you cannot keep them in view.

4. Are all the smoke detectors in your home working?

   Smoke detectors help save lives. Make sure that each detector has a working battery in it at all times.

5. Do you have a fire escape route that you practice regularly with your children?

   A planned escape route can help your children get out of your home quickly if fire breaks out. It's also a good idea to designate an outside meeting place.

Guns

1. Do you keep a gun in your home?

    If you do, seriously consider getting rid of it. If you decide to keep a gun, store it unloaded and in a locked location. Store ammunition separately in another locked location. These locations must be out of the reach of children.

Backyard

1. When you mow the lawn, clip a hedge with trimmers, or use other garden power equipment, is your child indoors?

    Power equipment can throw stones and other debris. Ride-on mowers pose a particular hazard for young children because the operator cannot see a child who is behind the mower. Keep children indoors until this type of yard work is finished.

2. Do you have a swimming pool, spa, or hot tub in the backyard?

    Young children are at risk of drowning in water, no matter the source. Install a fence with a locking gate around a pool, hot tub, or spa. Check the fence to make sure it remains sturdy and in good repair. Do not leave out buckets or other containers that can collect rainwater in the yard.

3. Do you know CPR?

    You may not always be able to prevent your child from getting into water when you are not present to supervise. Time is critical to rescue a child from drowning. Learn CPR: it can make a difference.

8

🌿 Safety, Room by Room

Homes differ immensely in their layout, furnishings, and uses, but most homes have a few features in common, such as a kitchen or cooking area, one or more bedrooms, and a bathroom. In these rooms and others, children may come across any number of hazards, so parents and caregivers have the responsibility to eliminate or minimize these hazards as much as possible. In the last chapter, I discussed common injury hazards for children in and around the home. In this chapter, I take you through specific rooms to identify hazards and how you can best address them to keep your children safe.

What's Cooking? Safety in the Kitchen

For many families, the kitchen functions as much more than simply a place to prepare and eat food. It may also serve as a family room, study, laundry room, and storage room. With so many uses, kitchens are bound to contain multiple hazards for children. According to a 2002 study, parents believe that it is generally unsafe for children younger than six years to be alone in the kitchen. Parents and caregivers recognize that kitchens contain numerous and varied hazards —mechanical, thermal, electrical, and chemical. Let's look at each of these hazards in turn.

Mechanical Hazards in the Kitchen

Mechanical hazards involve an object that physically interacts with a child so as to pose a risk of injury. Mechanical hazards in the kitchen and their possible consequences include

a closing drawer that pinches fingers
a sharp-edged knife that cuts a hand

a shattered glass dinner plate that punctures a cheek
a stool that a child falls from

The typical kitchen is full of equipment and utensils that present mechanical hazards, including knives, choppers, blenders, can and bottle openers, scissors, graters, and metal lids. The injuries that result from these hazards include cuts, punctures, bruises, and amputation.

You can reduce the risk of your child's being injured by common kitchen equipment and objects in several ways:

- Store knives and other sharp utensils in higher rather than lower drawers.
- Do not cut, chop, slice, or perform other similar tasks while holding a child or while using a surface within a child's reach.
- When you finish using sharp utensils, put them away immediately.
- Immediately throw away metal lids and pop-tops in a covered trashcan.
- Unplug blenders, mixers, choppers, and similar electrical appliances when not in use. Unplugging an appliance is the only way to guarantee that it won't start unintentionally.

When young children want to be kitchen "helpers," assign them tasks that will not bring them close to sharp items. For example, don't allow young children to place food in a blender or to hold items steady on a chopping board. Instead, you could ask them to stir a bowl of ingredients with a wooden spoon, crush crackers or cookies in a bag, or arrange salad ingredients on a plate. As children get older (older than eight years), teach them how to use cutting tools correctly. Safe Kids recommends that children be at least ten years old before being allowed to use appliances like blenders and microwaves. Even then, children should use appliances only under direct supervision.

Children frequently fall and injure themselves. While you cannot easily keep children who are already walking from falling, you can prevent falls for infants in carriers. Injury data tell us that infants often fall from heights while in their carriers, probably because adults find it convenient to place a carrier on top of a counter, table, or other elevated surface, especially for feeding. An infant's movements can cause a carrier to "walk" or slide over the surface and fall off. Newer carriers are required to be slip resistant—an acknowledgment by industry that some adults will continue to put carriers on elevated surfaces. An excellent place to put an infant in her carrier is on the floor,

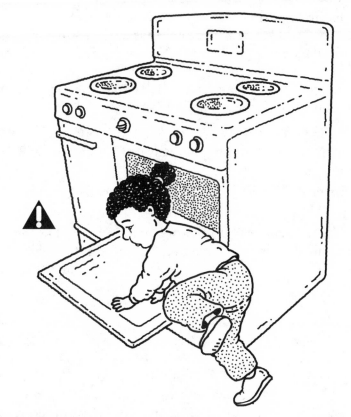

because she won't be able to fall anywhere. However, if you put an infant and carrier on the kitchen floor, be sure they are not near other kitchen hazards. Babies in carriers on the floor have been scalded when hot liquids have spilled from countertops.

Children have been known to sit on or climb onto open oven doors, and as a result, the entire stove can tip over. To prevent a stove from tipping over in this way, it should be bolted in place. A label on the oven door of newer models warns of this hazard, and a new stove also comes with hardware for securing it to the floor. In addition to being harmed by the stove itself as it tips over, children can be scalded when pots on the stovetop fall off as the stove tips. Hot liquid or food cascades down on them, usually burning a large area of the body.

Thermal Hazards in the Kitchen

Thermal hazards pose an injury risk because of their temperature. Although both hot and cold temperatures fall into this hazard category, thermal hazards in kitchens usually involve hot temperatures that cause burn or scald injuries. The kitchen is obviously one of the main locations in the home where thermal injuries occur, because cooking involves heat or open flames. A hot stove, a hot pan, and hot food or liquid are all sources of potential thermal injury. Thermal hazards and their consequences include such things as

- a hot cookie sheet that burns fingers or a hand when touched
- hot food or liquid, most commonly hot water, that spills and scalds a part of the body
- open flames or hot electrical coils that can cause clothing to catch on fire

Kitchen-related contact burns most often involve the fingers or hand and usually are not serious. A child's reflex action is to pull away from

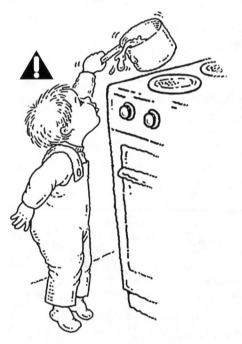

a hot surface, which minimizes the time of contact. However, when hot liquids spill onto a child, he cannot just pull away. Spills often occur on clothing, which then adheres to the skin. Children do not know enough to get out of clothing drenched by a hot liquid; they tend to cry and wait for someone to help them. The longer the contact time of the hot liquid and wet clothing on a child's body, the more severe the scald injury is likely to be. Scald injuries are particularly devastating because even a small amount of liquid can cover a large area of a child's body. Scalds often require hospitalization and surgery for skin grafting. Both skin grafting and scarring can have long-term physical and psychological effects.

The most common scenario in which a child is scalded occurs when a one-year-old (twelve to twenty-three months) reaches up and pulls a pot of hot water from the stovetop. Boys are more likely than girls to pull pans off the stove. In other situations, children, especially toddlers, are scalded when they

- reach across a table and overturn a container of hot food or liquid

- tug on the tail of a tablecloth and pull down cups or bowls of hot liquid, especially coffee and tea
- tug on appliance cords that hang over the edge of countertops and pull down the appliance (for example, a deep fryer) and its contents

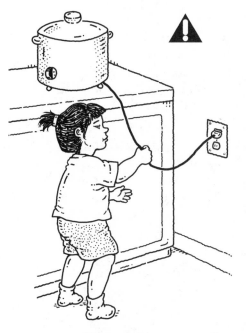

Children sitting in your lap while you drink hot liquids are also at risk for scalds. Sudden movements can cause you to spill hot liquid onto the child. The child may also put his fingers into your cup or overturn the cup. And as mentioned above, children can also be scalded if they sit or climb on an open oven door and cause pots of hot food or liquid on the stovetop to fall onto them.

Young children can reach farther than you might think, and they are determined climbers. So to reduce the risk of scalds to younger children, get into the habit of doing the following things while working in the kitchen:

- Keep children away from the stove and countertops when you are cooking.
- Whenever possible, use the rear burners. Turn cookware handles toward the back of the stove. Even a one-year-old can reach the front burners from a standing position.
- Don't hold a child in your arms while you are cooking, because she can reach into pots, grab utensils, get splashed, and overturn pots.
- Don't eat or drink hot foods and liquids while holding a child in your arms or lap.
- Forgo the use of placemats and tablecloths until your children get older.
- Don't give children more mobility than they need—don't put your infant in a walker in the kitchen, for example. When young children need to be in the kitchen with you, try to create a minienvironment especially for them. Position a highchair, playpen, or infant carrier so that your child cannot reach

the stove, counters, or hazardous objects and so that dangerous items cannot fall onto the child.

Older children, aged three to five years, are scalded less often than
younger children are, and they tend to be scalded in different ways.
Scalds suffered by these older children may happen when they are running and collide with someone carrying a pot of hot water or food,
or they knock something off a stove with another item, like a toy baseball bat. The best way to minimize the scalding risk to this age group
is to explain to children why they should not run and play games in
the kitchen. And each time you move a pot of hot food or liquid from
one location to another, glance around to see where your children are.

Microwave ovens are so easy to use that you might think a five-
year-old can make her own popcorn or lunch. Remember, though,
that microwaves heat both the food and the dish and that children do
not have the skill to handle hot foods and containers appropriately.
Wait until children are nine or ten years old before you allow them to
use the microwave, and supervise them whenever they do.

People frequently store matches and lighters in the kitchen, often
in a drawer or a high cabinet. Young children, especially three- to five-
year-olds, tend to be fascinated by fire. At this age, children typically
try to use lighters to make play fires, while children older than five
years usually create play fires with matches. Children playing with fire
account for only 5 percent of residential fires, yet such fires cause 40
percent of residential fire-related deaths among children. Although
children may find lighters or matches in the kitchen, more than half
of all child play fires in homes begin in a bedroom. Disposable, novelty, and multipurpose lighters must adhere to child-resistance regulations, but don't assume that these lighters are childproof. Some children younger than five years may be able to operate child-resistant
lighters.

Remember that children like to imitate you—in fact, much of their
learning occurs through imitation. Some young children who started
play fires had watched adults use a multipurpose lighter to light a pilot light or a barbecue. Avoid doing something in front of children if
the action could put them at risk when they try to repeat it. If you
must perform a potentially hazardous task in their presence, then use
the opportunity to teach them about avoiding the risk. Keep in mind,
however, that only older children can fully comprehend information
about hazards and risks. Children don't really understand the danger
of fire until they are about nine years old.

Electrical Hazards in the Kitchen

Today most U.S. kitchens are equipped with a coffeemaker, a toaster, a blender, and several other small electrical appliances. With electrical equipment comes the potential for electric shock. Electric shocks from kitchen equipment are rare these days, probably because most, if not all, small electrical appliances meet safety standards that address shock hazards. Nevertheless, it is good practice to unplug any small electrical appliances that are not in use and to keep cords out of children's reach. When appliances are in use, make sure the cord does not dangle over the edge of the counter, because, as mentioned in the thermal hazards section, one tug on a cord can land the entire appliance and its contents on a child. It's also best to keep children from using electrical appliances with a heating element, like a toaster, until they are at least eight years old.

Chemical Hazards in the Kitchen

Kitchens often house batteries and household chemicals (cleaners, bleaches, and the like), including poisonous, irritant, caustic, and flam-

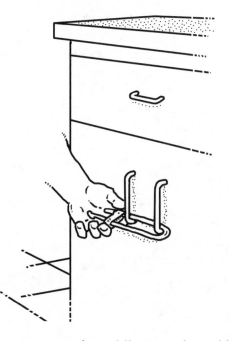

mable materials. Children younger than five years, and especially one- to three-year-olds, are at the highest risk of chemical ingestion and poisoning. In 2002, poison control centers received reports of more than 1.2 million unintentional poisonings among children five years and younger. About 60 percent of the products involved were nonpharmaceuticals, such as cleaning substances, cosmetics, pesticides, and poisonous plants, and 40 percent were pharmaceuticals.

Many chemical products come in child-resistant packaging. Keep them that way. Don't be tempted to transfer products into a non–child-resistant container for convenience. Use cabinet locks to keep chemical storage areas out of a toddler's reach, and keep handy the phone number of a local poison control center. The U.S. National Poison Control Hotline can be reached at 1-800-222-1222.

Note that the American Academy of Pediatrics no longer recommends syrup of ipecac as a home treatment for poisoning. The recommendation changed because research showed no benefit for children treated with ipecac. Most emergency departments have also stopped using ipecac in favor of activated charcoal, which is more effective.

❦ Key Actions to Prevent Injuries in the Kitchen

Although it may require some planning, you can simultaneously work in your kitchen and keep your children safe from kitchen hazards.

1. Store and use sharp equipment and utensils well away from children.
2. Store matches, lighters, batteries, and chemical products in locked cabinets or other locations out of children's reach.
3. Unplug appliances when not in use, keep cords from dangling over countertops, and don't allow your child to use an electric appliance until she is at least eight or nine years old, and then only under your supervision.
4. Place infants and young children in a confined space, like a high chair or playpen, located where they will not be able to reach hazards and nothing can fall on them. Explain to older children the need to treat the kitchen with respect, not as a playroom.
5. Have your stove bolted down, use back burners on the stovetop, and if you use front burners, turn pan handles toward the back of the stove.
6. Avoid using tablecloths and placemats. Don't hold children or sit them in your lap when you are working with or consuming hot foods and liquids.
7. Keep emergency phone numbers in an easily accessible location, such as taped inside a cabinet door.

Spending Time Together: Safety in the Living or Family Room

Aside from being in the kitchen, many families spend a lot of their indoor time together in a living room or family room. Common items in living and family rooms are sofas, chairs, tables, fireplaces, rugs, decorative items, pillows, TVs, stereo equipment, bookshelves, ceiling fans, and fish tanks. People tend to view these items as being fairly safe; yet many injuries occur in living and family rooms. Young children, especially one- to three-year-olds, often fall and strike furniture—in particular the corner of a coffee table. Children commonly injure their face and eyes when they fall against furniture. Because it is hard to control falls, your best alternative is to buy protective covers for corners. A child may still fall and injure herself, but with a corner protector the injury should not be as severe as it might be otherwise.

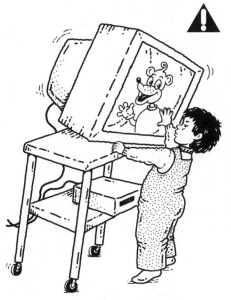

Children are curious explorers, and this behavior does not stop in the living or family room. As they try to move objects or clamber up, onto, and over furniture, children can easily pull down items or topple things over. Children have died as a result of being struck by falling TVs and bookcases. Incidents have also occurred with fish tanks, tables, and other electronic equipment. To reduce the risk of these types of injury,

- secure bookcases to the wall
- place TVs on stable surfaces, out of young children's reach
- store long, dangling electrical cords after use
- keep items that belong to children or are particularly attractive to them within their easy reach so they do not have to climb to get them.

Other common hazards in a living or family room are soft furniture, fireplaces, and electrical outlets. Sofas and soft chairs are hazardous sleep locations for an infant, because he can suffocate on pillows, between seat cushions, or between a seat cushion and the side of the sofa or chair. Always place an infant in his crib to sleep. Sofas and soft chairs are also unstable surfaces for an infant in a carrier. The carrier can overturn and trap the baby between the carrier and sofa or chair, where he may suffocate.

Fireplaces and woodstoves are attractive with their bright dancing flames, but they become incredibly hot very quickly. Securely attach protective screens to reduce the risk of a child's falling onto or touching a hot unit and being burned.

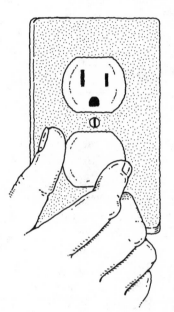

Electrical outlets are intriguing for children who have the manual skills to hold objects and poke them into holes. The risk of electric shock is serious, so cover all unused electrical outlets with safety plugs.

Several other hazards are less common and less recognized, but they are no less real and you should be aware of them. When an adult lifts a baby toward the ceiling, the child can be bumped into a doorway, a beam, or fan blades. These bumps can result in injuries such as bruises and cuts to the head and face. Tossing babies upward is also associated with retinal hemorrhage (bleeding at the back of the eyeball). It's best to keep an infant on the ground or on your lap, where you can safely interact and play with her. Finally, bean bag chairs with zippers were involved in five suffocation deaths between 1973 and 1995. Children enjoyed unzipping and getting inside the chairs—one child pretended to be in a space capsule. Since 1998, a safety standard for bean bag chairs has required manufacturers to make the zippers inoperable or lockable.

✦ Key Actions to Prevent Injuries in the Living or Family Room

Keep your children safe in the living or family room in the following ways.

1. Place protective corners on coffee tables and other furniture with sharp corners, or arrange furniture so children won't fall against it.
2. Secure heavy items, such as bookcases, TVs, and fish tanks, so that children can't knock them over.
3. Install protective screens around fireplaces and woodstoves.
4. Insert safety plugs in unused electrical outlets, and keep electrical cords where they can't be tripped over.
5. Put infants to sleep in a crib, not on a sofa or soft chair. Place an infant carrier on the floor, not on a sofa or soft chair.

Sleepy Time: Safety in the Bedroom

As I mentioned earlier, a child's bedroom tends to have furniture and products manufactured in accordance with child safety standards. For information about infants' and children's sleeping areas, refer back to Chapter 2 on sleeping. The following section deals with the parents' bedroom or another bedroom in a house.

Parents often bring their infant into their bedroom to nurse or to sleep. Unfortunately, doing this leads to the possibility of infant suffocation, the primary hazard of the parents' bedroom. Most frequently, infants suffocate because they are trapped between an adult bed and the wall. Three- to six-month-old infants are at the highest risk of getting trapped and suffocating in this way. Infants may also become trapped in other locations on an adult bed, including between the headboard and mattress, between the mattress and frame, and between the footboard and mattress. Bedding and pillows can cover an infant's face or create a pocket of stale air, resulting in suffocation. Avoid using pillows as props or barriers with an infant. And finally, sometimes an infant has suffocated when a parent rolls onto or against him. Babies younger than three months are at highest risk for this particular pattern of suffocation.

Parents' bedrooms and the bedrooms of older children may have several additional hazards for infants and young children:

- Water beds and infants don't go together. In fact, an infant should never be placed on a water bed, because the heat of a heated bed can contribute to hyperthermia (excessive heat), and the surface's tendency to mold around an infant's body can cause suffocation, regardless of whether the water bed is heated.
- Avoid placing a baby in a carrier on top of a bed. The carrier can overturn on the mattress, in the same way as on sofas and soft chairs, and trap and suffocate the baby.
- Children can and will climb into all sorts of spaces, including hope chests. Children have suffocated in hope chests that lock automatically.
- Children climb up and pull on dresser drawers, and this may tip the dresser over. A child trapped beneath a dresser may be physically injured from its impact and weight and may also suffocate if the dresser compresses her chest. When you fill drawers, place heavier items in the bottom ones to help stabi-

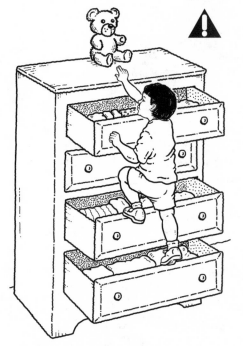

lize the dresser and reduce the risk of its tipping over.

- Medications are often kept on bedside tables or in dresser drawers. Keep all medications, including nonprescription medications, out of children's reach.
- Older siblings may have age-appropriate toys, TVs, video games, or other items in their bedroom that may pose injury risks to a younger child. Keep younger children out of older children's bedrooms, and teach older children to keep their possessions out of younger children's reach.

❧ Key Actions to Prevent Injuries in the Bedroom

Your infant or child can safely be in your bedroom if you follow certain precautions.

1. Don't bring your infant into your bed when you plan to sleep yourself. Nurse her and then return her to her crib when you are ready to sleep.
2. Keep pillows and soft bedding away from an infant, and never put an infant on a water bed.
3. Never put an infant in his carrier on a bed.
4. Stabilize dressers so that they won't tip over, and lock hope chests and other similar furniture so that children can't climb inside.
5. Keep medications out of children's reach.
6. Decide how you will keep a young child safe from toys and other items in an older child's bedroom.

Beyond Bathtubs: Safety in the Bathroom

Bathrooms contain an obvious hazard—water in the bathtub—which I discussed in detail in Chapter 3 and will mention again, more briefly, here. There are, however, several other hazards found in bathrooms, including toilets, pharmaceuticals and beauty products, and electrical appliances.

The injuries that occur in bathtubs are drowning and scalding. A child can drown quickly and in very little water—a matter of only a few inches—so never leave a child unattended in the tub, not even for a moment. Don't be fooled that a young child is safe in the tub with an older sibling present. The young child needs your constant supervision. A bath seat is not a babysitter, either, and does not guarantee that a child will be safe if you leave to answer the phone, to check on another child, or to fetch the shampoo you forgot. Stay with a child for the entire time that she is in the tub. About half of infant drownings occur in a bathtub.

Scalding, a second hazard with tubs, typically occurs after a child in the tub or a sibling outside it turns on the hot water tap. Young children sitting in very hot water do not know to get out of it, even if they are physically capable of climbing out. Instead, they stay in the hot water until they are rescued, with the result that scalds can be quite severe.

Curious toddlers will bend over to look and reach into toilet bowls. If they lose their balance and fall in head first, they cannot get out, and they drown in the toilet water. Keep the door to the bathroom closed, use a baby gate at its entrance, or put a lock on the toilet lid.

Most people store medicines, beauty and health products, and other potentially poisonous substances in the bathroom. Store these products out of children's reach. When you use a product, be sure to properly resecure the child-resistant closure, and leave products in their child-resistant containers rather than transferring them to an ordinary container. Keep handy the National Poison Control Center's phone number: 1-800-222-1222.

Finally, remember that an appliance that is turned off but still plugged in can carry electricity and give an electric shock if it's dropped into water. Unplug hairdryers and other small appliances when they're not in use, and position appliances so that they can't fall or be pulled into water when you are using them.

⌁ Key Actions to Prevent Injuries in the Bathroom

Any bathroom contains several hazards, but with your watchfulness, your children will be safe while in the bathroom.

1. Stay with a bathing child at all times. Bring everything you need into the bathroom, and ignore distractions outside the room.
2. Test the temperature of bathwater with a thermometer before placing a child into the water.
3. Keep the door to the bathroom closed, use a baby gate at its entrance, or put a lock on the toilet seat lid.
4. Keep all medications, beauty products, and other substances out of children's reach.
5. Use electrical appliances away from water, and when you are done, unplug and store them out of children's reach.

Clean Clothes: Safety in the Laundry Room

The area with your laundry machines, whether it be an entire room, a closet, or simply one corner of another room, contains several hazards for infants and young children. It is best not to take children into the laundry area with you. Laundry areas usually have detergent, bleach, and similar products, all of which can be poisonous if ingested. Bleach and some other cleaners are also skin irritants and can cause serious problems if they come into contact with the eyes. Store all laundry products out of children's reach.

A less obvious hazard in laundry areas, but one that accounts for about half of washer/dryer-related injuries to children five years and younger, is a fall from a height. Sometimes parents have set an infant in a carrier or car seat on top of a washer or dryer and the child has fallen to the floor in the carrier, commonly suffering head and face injuries. Older children have fallen after climbing onto a washer or dryer.

❦ Key Actions to Prevent Injuries in the Laundry Room

Ideally, you will not take children into the laundry area with you. If you must, or if your laundry area is part of a common space like the kitchen, then follow these precautions to keep children safe.

1. Place all detergents and other laundry products out of your child's reach.
2. Place your infant in his carrier on the floor, away from the appliances and shelving.

3. Don't allow older children to climb onto or sit on top of a washer or dryer.

Storing Stuff: Safety in Sheds, Basements, and Garages

Garden equipment, carpentry tools, paint and varnish, a hot water tank, a car—all such belongings need to be kept somewhere. Many households keep all of these items, plus an assortment of others, in a shed, the basement, or a garage. These rooms may contain outdoor equipment, such as lawn mowers and hedge trimmers; hand tools, including drills, hammers, and screwdrivers; power tools, such as table saws and belt sanders; and flammable or toxic products, like glues and paint thinners. The basement usually houses the water heater and the furnace as well.

Outdoor equipment, tools, home repair products, and basement appliances are not suitable for young children to be in contact with, so garages, sheds, and basements should be completely off limits to children younger than five years. There are simply too many hazardous items present. You can restrict children's access, depending on their age and abilities, with baby gates, closed doors, or locked doors. Some power tools come with child-resistant safety locks. Use these locks, even though you keep the equipment in a location that your child can't access.

The basement, or wherever a gas furnace or gas water heater is located, can be the place where a house fire begins. Gas furnaces and water heaters have a pilot light—an open flame that can ignite the vapors of flammable products and cause an explosion and a fire. If you must store flammables in the same area as a gas furnace or water heater, place the flammable substances as far away from the gas appliances as possible, and keep the flammables in tightly sealed containers. Never store gasoline anywhere inside a house. When you use flammable products, use them with plenty of ventilation so the fumes and vapors will dissipate.

Garage doors can be deadly if they trap a child as they close. Since 1993, however, garage doors must be manufactured with an auto-reverse function that takes effect within two seconds of contacting an obstruction. To reduce the likelihood that children will play with a garage door, install the garage-door control device out of children's reach, and lock the remote control in your car's glove compartment. Also, keep your car locked to prevent children from playing in the trunk or passenger area of the car.

❦ Key Actions to Prevent Injuries in Sheds, Basements, and Garages

Keep your child safe from the equipment, products, and appliances found in a shed, basement, or garage in the following ways.

1. Use baby gates, closed doors, or locks to prevent your child from entering the shed, basement, and garage.
2. Use child-resistant safety locks, if they are provided, on power equipment.
3. Store flammable products well away from ignition sources, such as pilot lights.
4. Keep the remote control for a garage door away from children, and always lock your car.

One and Two and . . . : Safety in the Exercise Room

Some people are dedicated to their exercise routines, and other people find it difficult to squeeze enough time from a day to even contemplate exercise. Parents of young children may get plenty of exercise simply keeping up with their active youngsters! Nonetheless, many people find it convenient to use exercise equipment, like a treadmill, a stationary bike, or weights, at home. Because of moving parts and the weight and instability of some pieces of equipment, all exercise equipment should be kept in an area that young children cannot access.

Treadmills, in particular, are dangerous for young children. About one-third of all treadmill-related injuries from 1995 to 2000 involved children five years and younger, with the average age for injury being three years. Most of these children received friction burns from contact with the moving surface or became trapped between the conveyor belt and the machine's base. Injuries sustained in these incidents usually involved the arm, forearm, wrist, hand, or fingers. Such injuries can be serious enough to require hospitalization, surgery, and rehabilitation treatment with a physical therapist. Surgery can leave scars that a child will have for the rest of her life. Most of the treadmill injuries reported during the 1995–2000 period occurred while a parent was using the equipment, so keep in mind that you should exercise when your children are elsewhere or when your infant is safely contained within a playpen.

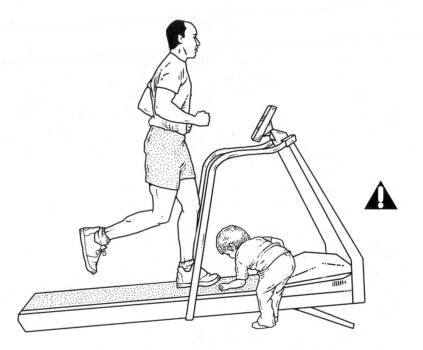

⫓ Key Actions to Prevent Injuries in the Exercise Room

Exercise is good for you, but the equipment you use can be hazardous to your child. Keep your child safe from injuries in the following ways.

1. Use baby gates or closed doors to keep your child out of the exercise room.
2. Use exercise equipment when your child is being looked after by someone else. If your infant or toddler must be in the room with you, have him in a carrier or playpen placed well away from the equipment.

Summing Up

Young children will have access to many areas of your home and to household products not intended for them or designed with their safety in mind. Your attentiveness is necessary to keep children protected from hazardous products and other risks that are present throughout your home. Your key to exercising caution is to understand and recognize possible injury hazards. Try to think about each room in your home from a child's viewpoint—get down on your hands and knees, if necessary, and take a look around. Then move, secure, or store items that could injure your child. Remember, too, that as your child grows and develops, she will be able to reach items that she couldn't reach before, or she may become interested in items that didn't interest her before.

Wander into each room in your home while you read the safety checklist below. My guess is that you'll find several things you're already doing correctly and a few things that need to be changed. For your child's safety, for your peace of mind, and for your family's well-being, create the best possible environment for your child's early years of life. It will be well worth it.

Room-by-Room Safety Checklist

Go through the following room-by-room checklist as you consider each room in your home.

Kitchen

1. Do you store and use sharp equipment and utensils well away from your child?

   Remember that the hand is quicker than the eye, and a child can grab a sharp edge before you can stop him. Store sharp utensils where children cannot reach them, or put a child lock on the drawer or door.

2. Is your stove bolted down?

   Children sit and climb on open oven doors. If the stove is not bolted down, it can tip over onto a child.

3. What do you do to reduce the risk that your toddler will be scalded?

   Try to use back burners on the stovetop, and turn pan handles toward the back of the stove. Appliance cords are inviting to pull on, so keep them from dangling over countertops. Avoid using tablecloths and placemats until your child is much older. Do not hold your child in your arms while you are cooking or eating; instead, place her in her high chair, playpen, or carrier, well away from hazards.

4. Where do you store matches or lighters?

   Children are enthralled by fire, and many experiment with it. Store matches and lighters well out of children's reach, re-

membering that children can and do climb when they are determined to find something.

5. Where do you store batteries, household cleaners, and other
   chemical products?

   Poisoning is a real risk with many of the products that people tend to keep under the kitchen sink. If you have a toddler,
   use child locks on cabinets that contain chemical products.
   Keep the National Poison Control phone number (1-800-
   222-1222) and other emergency phone numbers in an easily
   accessible location, such as inside a cabinet door.

6. Do you unplug small appliances when they are not in use?

   Keeping appliances unplugged will ensure that your young
   child cannot start them.

7. Do you allow your child to cook or use the microwave?

   These tasks are too risky for young children. Instead, give
   them kitchen tasks that do not involve heat or hot surfaces.
   Only when children are eight or nine years old can they begin to use kitchen appliances, and then only under your direct supervision.

Living Room or Family Room

1. If your child is three years or younger, do you have protective
   corners on the coffee table?

   Coffee tables are often in the way of children, especially
   climbing and running toddlers, who inevitably fall onto a corner of the coffee table. While you may not be able to stop the
   fall, you can soften it and reduce the severity of injury by using corner protectors.

2. Is the TV placed securely?

   The TV should be out of reach and on a stable stand to
   minimize the risk of tip-over. If you have a video game con-
   sole connected to the TV, wrap up the cords and put them out
   of reach after use, so your youngster cannot pull on them.

3. Are bookcases or other storage units secured to the wall?

   Children can climb onto bookcases and other types of storage units and cause them to tip over. Fasten bookcases and
   storage units to the wall.

4. If you have a fireplace or woodstove, is there a protective
   screen around it?

Children are attracted to fire, yet they don't understand the danger. A screen can effectively separate your child from the heat and flames.

5. Are there any unused electrical outlets in your home?

Cover unused electrical outlets with safety plugs so that your child won't put his fingers or other objects into the socket.

6. Have you put your baby to sleep on the sofa, or have you placed the baby in her carrier on the sofa or a soft chair?

Soft surfaces increase the risk of tip-over for carriers and of suffocation for babies. Put your baby to sleep in a crib, not on a sofa or soft chair, and place her in her carrier on the floor, not on a sofa or soft chair.

Bedroom

Also review the Sleep Safely Checklist in Chapter 2.

1. Do you bring your baby into your bed?

For the reasons I have discussed, an adult bed is not a safe place for an infant to spend the night. Nurse and play with your baby in your bed, but return him to his crib when you are ready to sleep. If you insist on keeping your baby with you all night, remove the mattress from the bed frame and place it on the floor, away from the wall. Remove pillows and soft bedding.

2. Do you have a hope chest or similar storage furniture in your room?

Children like to hide in enclosed spaces. Unfortunately, they can suffocate inside. Be sure that hope chests and other storage furnishings are locked or not accessible to your child.

3. Where do you keep medications?

For convenience many of us keep medications in or on a bedside table, but children easily find them there. Keep medications in their child-resistant containers, and store them out of your child's reach.

4. Can your younger children enter your older children's bedrooms?

It can be a challenge to keep young children away from older children's belongings and playthings. You can teach your older children about the hazards their possessions might pose for younger children, but it may be easier to try to make their bedrooms inaccessible by use of, for example, safety doorknob covers.

Bathroom

Also review the Bathe Safely Checklist in Chapter 3.

1. Does the toilet lid have a lock?

    Toddlers can drown in a toilet. Install a lock on the toilet seat lid, set up a baby gate at the bathroom entrance, or keep the bathroom door closed.

2. Do you keep all medications, beauty products, and other substances out of your child's reach?

    Many of these products can be attractive and poisonous for a child. Keep them out of your child's reach, and always secure any child-resistant closures.

3. Do you unplug and store electrical appliances that are not in use?

    Electricity and water are a dangerous mix. Plugged-in appliances still have electric current in them, even if they are in the "off" position. When you are finished with them, unplug and store hair dryers, shavers, and any other small appliances you use in the bathroom.

4. To what temperature is your hot water heater set?

    Scalds can be devastating injuries. Keep your whole family safe from bath or shower scalds by maintaining a moderate temperature setting on the water heater (about 120° F).

Laundry Room

1. Do you keep detergents and all other laundry products in their original containers and out of your child's reach?

    Many laundry products are poisonous or are eye and respiratory irritants. Keep them out of your child's reach and in their original containers.

2. If you take your infant into the laundry area in a carrier, do you place the carrier on the floor?

    Set your infant in her carrier on the floor, not on top of the washer or dryer. A number of infants have been hurt by falling in their carrier off a washer or dryer.

Shed, Basement, and Garage

1. Can your child get into a shed, basement, or garage without you?

   These areas of your home tend to be full of products that are dangerous. It is best to keep them locked.
2. Do any tools in your shed, basement, or garage have child-resistant features?

   Some power tools have safety features that prevent accidental startup by children. If any of your tools has a safety feature, use it.
3. If you have flammable products in the basement, are they tightly capped and stored well away from ignition sources, such as pilot lights?

   Flammables and their vapors can catch fire or explode if they come in contact with an open flame or spark. Store these products as far away as you can from ignition sources, like your gas water heater and furnace, and keep them tightly capped so vapors do not escape.
4. Where do you keep the remote control for the garage door?

   To keep children from playing with the garage door, install the interior control unit out of a child's reach, and keep the remote control locked in your car's glove compartment. Keep the car locked as well.

Exercise Room

1. If you have an exercise room or area, can your child get to the equipment?

   Use baby gates or closed doors to keep your child out of the exercise room.
2. Where is your child while you exercise?

   Use exercise equipment when your child is napping or being looked after by someone else. If your infant must be in the room with you, have him in a carrier or playpen placed where he cannot touch the equipment.

Appendix

INJURY PREVENTION SUMMARY CHARTS

CHART 1
SLEEPING

Injury	Age at Highest Risk*	How to Prevent Injury
Suffocation		
Covering the nose/mouth	birth to 6 months	Empty crib of all toys and stuffed animals for sleeping Do not place blankets, quilts, comforters, or pillows in crib Keep plastic bags away from crib
Wedging	3 to 6 months	Place infant on her back in crib for sleeping Use only mattress that came with crib, because correct mattress fit is critical Avoid placing baby on adult bed or sofa to sleep
Tilted surfaces	birth to 6 months	Keep sleep surface level; be sure any swinging product comes to rest level Check that bassinet legs are locked in place
Overlying	birth to 2 months	Put baby to sleep alone (not with a sibling) in crib or bassinet Do not take baby into your bed for sleeping through the night
Hanging and strangling		
Hanging	7 months to 3 years	Position crib away from windows Make sure window coverings have no loops Do not put necklaces or any other loops around child's neck Do not put hooded clothing on child Check that crib endpost (finial) height is less than 0.06 (approximately 1/16) inch above headboard and footboard
Strangling	7 to 12 months	Do not allow toys with ribbons, strings, or cords in crib Do not allow child to sleep with clothing that has ribbons, strings, or cords

CHART 1 SLEEPING
Continued

Injury	Age at Highest Risk*	How to Prevent Injury
Postural strangling	5 to 9 months	Remove crib gyms from crib when infant reaches 5 months of age or can push up on hands and knees Remove toys that attach to the side of the crib by ties when infant reaches 5 months of age or can push up on hands and knees
Related to trapping	12 to 24 months	Securely lock all latches on playpens and other collapsible items
Compression and trapping		
Within crib	3 to 12 months	Check crib integrity, especially for loose or missing bolts or slats Check mattress supports for integrity; make sure mattress does not sag in any corner
Between crib and furniture	12 to 24 months	Do not place crib adjacent to other furniture
In mesh-sided playpens	birth to 6 months	Make sure mesh-sided playpen sides are fully erect
In toddler beds	2 to 4 years	Check that spacing between guard rails is less than 2.7 (approximately 2¾) inches
In bunk beds	4 to 5 years (and older)	Do not allow children younger than 6 years on upper bunk Check that spacing between mattress and frame is less than 3½ inches
Positional asphyxia	7 to 11 months	Keep hampers, pails, and containers away from where baby sleeps
Rebreathing	birth to 6 months	Put baby to sleep on her back Make sure mattress surface is firm

Continued

Chart 1 SLEEPING
Continued

Injury	Age at Highest Risk*	How to Prevent Injury
		Never put baby on top of quilt, comforter, pillow, or other soft bedding
Burns	all ages	Have children wear sleepwear or snug-fitting cotton and cotton blends to bed

*Children outside these age ranges can also suffer these kinds of injuries, but children in the age range given suffer them most often.

CHART 2
BATHING AND DRESSING

Injury	Age at Highest Risk*	How to Prevent Injury
Bathing		
Drowning	5 months to 2 years	Stay with child for entire bath time, even if you use a bath ring or bath seat Ignore distractions, like phone and doorbell Take all bathing needs into bathroom before you start child's bath
Scalding	1 to 2 years	Set hot water heater to deliver water no hotter than 125° F Test water temperature with bath thermometer Seat child facing away from faucets Stay with child for entire bath time
Electrocution	1 to 5 years	Unplug all electrical appliances when not in use Do not allow children to operate electrical appliances
Dressing		
Poisoning and aspiration	6 to 18 months	Keep lotions and creams, especially baby oil, out of baby's reach
Falls from changing table	4 to 12 months	Have all changing needs at hand Keep one hand on baby at all times
Choking on clothing accessories	6 months to 3 years	Check that buttons, snaps, and other attachments on clothing are securely attached
Strangling and hanging	10 months to 5 years	Make sure there are no ribbons or cords at neckline Do not put necklaces on child or tie any items around child's neck Do not tie pacifier around child's neck; use pacifier leash
Becoming trapped in moving parts	2 to 5 years	Avoid loose-fitting clothes and clothes with dangling cords

*Children outside these age ranges can also suffer these kinds of injuries, but children in the age range given suffer them most often.

CHART 3
EATING

Injury	Age at Highest Risk*	How to Prevent Injury
Choking	6 months to 4 years	Give children appropriate foods Avoid giving children younger than 5 years the following: rounded, slippery foods like hot dogs and grapes; nuts and popcorn; hard candy; hard raw vegetables, like celery and carrots; raisins; gobs of peanut butter Have children remain seated while eating Teach children to chew and swallow before speaking Do not have slightly older siblings feed younger ones Learn age-appropriate first aid for choking
Scalds and burns	birth to 2 years	Shake or stir well any heated foods to minimize hot spots Place feeding dishes out of child's reach Do not use tablecloths or placemats
Strangling and trapping	6 months to 3 years	Use high chair's safety restraint system Position tray table close against child Stay with child for entire feeding time
Falls	6 months to 2 years	Use high chair's safety restraint system Stay with child for entire feeding time Avoid placing infant carrier on an elevated surface; if you do, place carrier away from edges and keep a hand on it Position hook-on chair away from table legs and other push-off points Do not put a regular chair under the hook-on chair
Giving medications	all ages	Use an accurate dose-delivery method

*Children outside these age ranges can also suffer these kinds of injuries, but children in the age range given suffer them most often.

CHART 4
PLAYING

Injury	Age at Highest Risk*	How to Prevent Injury
Falls		
Indoor	12 months to 3 years	Cover edges of furniture, particularly coffee tables
		Secure shelving to wall
		Use baby gates at top and bottom of stairs
		Arrange furniture to discourage climbing onto counters, window sills, and other elevated areas
		Carpet play areas to soften ground-level falls; for indoor climbing equipment, install appropriate protective surfacing
		Keep children from walking and running with items in the mouth, especially pens and pencils
Outdoor	2 to 5 years (and older)	Have children wear helmets and other protective equipment (bike helmet, skating pads, etc.) appropriate to the activity
		Check depth of protective surfacing under playground equipment; mulch should be fluffy, at least 6 inches deep, and evenly spread out
Becoming tangled, hanging, and strangling		
On long cords or ribbons	10 to 18 months	Do not add string, cord, or ribbon to any toy
		Strings on toys should be shorter than 12 inches, unless it's a pull toy
On clothing drawstrings	2 to 5 years (and older)	No drawstrings at neckline of children's clothing
On other clothing, accessories	8 months to 5 years	Remove anything around the neck—necklace, scarf, bib, etc.—when children play

Continued

CHART 4 PLAYING
Continued

Injury	Age at Highest Risk*	How to Prevent Injury
On crib gyms	5 to 9 months	Remove crib gyms from crib when infant can push up on hands and knees or reaches 5 months of age, whichever comes first
On crib mobile strings	8 to 12 months	Install mobiles out of infant's reach Remove mobiles from crib when infant can push up on hands and knees or reaches 5 months of age, whichever comes first
Becoming trapped		
In an opening	2 to 5 years	Openings in play equipment should be smaller than 3½ inches *or* larger than 9 inches
In a collapsed product	8 months to 2 years	Fully lock latches on playpen and any other product in which child is placed
In a closed space	2 to 5 years	Make sure toy chest lid does not fall shut If you think toy chest lid is not safe, remove it completely If child is missing, check car trunk, coolers, hope chests, and other closed containers If you discard an appliance, always take the doors off
Choking		
On balloons	10 months to 3 years	Give children in this age range Mylar balloons, not latex Do not allow children through 8 years old to blow up latex balloons Throw away broken latex balloons immediately

CHART 4 PLAYING
Continued

Injury	Age at Highest Risk*	How to Prevent Injury
On small parts	1 to 2 years	Buy age-appropriate toys Keep older children's toys away from young children Check toys, especially those with magnetic components, to make sure they are not broken
On small balls and marbles	1 to 5 years	Make sure balls for children younger than 3 years are larger than 1¾ inches in diameter Do not give marbles to children younger than 5 years
On toy attachments	6 months to 2 years	Tug on attachments, like eyes, to make sure they are securely fastened Remove any pieces that become loose
Suffocation		
On oval-, cup-, or bowl-shaped items	8 months to 2 years	Avoid toys of this shape for this age group, unless toy has holes that prevent suction from forming, or unless item is smaller than 2½ inches or larger than 4 inches in diameter
Pinching, crushing, or shearing		
In folding toys	1 to 3 years	Make sure foldable items are fully open and locked in position
In moving parts	2 to 5 years	Avoid motorized (battery-operated) toys with moving parts for children younger than 4 years
Burns		
Sunburn	all ages	Limit time outdoors, especially between 10 a.m. and 4 p.m., when sun is brightest Apply sunscreen liberally and often

Continued

CHART 4 PLAYING
Continued

Injury	Age at Highest Risk*	How to Prevent Injury
		Cover up: brimmed hats, cotton clothing, long sleeves
		Keep infants under 6 months old out of direct sun
On outdoor play equipment	1 to 5 years	If play area is sunny, touch equipment, especially slides, before allowing children on
On battery-operated toys	birth to 5 years	Check batteries often to make sure they are not leaking
		Replace batteries when needed, using all the same type of battery
		Be sure to insert batteries in correct orientation
		Remove batteries when item will not be used for a month or more
Hearing damage		
From loud toys	birth to 2 years	Do not create loud noise close to child's ear
		Choose toys that make soft, soothing sounds

*Children outside these age ranges can also suffer these kinds of injuries, but children in the age range given suffer them most often.

CHART 5
TRAVEL

Injury	Age at Highest Risk*	How to Prevent Injury
Vehicle: Car seats		
Car crash	all ages	Make sure children younger than 12 years ride in the back seat
		Make sure each child is secured in appropriate car seat or booster seat
		Make sure car seat or booster seat is installed correctly (see seat instructions)
		Make sure restraint straps are located correctly on child's body (see seat instructions)
		If a car seat has been involved in a crash, replace it
		Do not buy a used car seat unless you are sure of its history
Strangling	1 to 2 years	Make sure restraint is correctly secured
		Do not leave child alone in vehicle
Vehicle: Other		
Hyperthermia	birth to 5 years	Do not leave children alone in vehicle, especially a closed vehicle in the summer months
Inadvertent starting	2 to 5 years	Do not leave children alone in vehicle
		Take keys with you; store keys out of children's reach
Window or door trapping	2 to 5 years	Turn off back seat controls for windows
		Engage child locks for rear doors
Driveway run-over	1 to 4 years	Know where your children are before you pull out of driveway
Trunk trapping	2 to 5 years	Keep vehicle locked at home
Carriers and strollers		
Pinching and shearing	1 to 2 years	Fully open and lock carriages and strollers

Continued

CHART 5 TRAVEL
Continued

Injury	Age at Highest Risk*	How to Prevent Injury
Falls	1 to 3 years	Use restraint straps
Tip-over	birth to 3 years	Do not load rear of carriage or stroller with purchases or heavy bags
Trapping	8 months to 2 years	Use restraint straps Put leg rest up when child is sleeping Keep sleeping child in view
Infant carriers		
Falls	birth to 8 months	Routinely check carrier handles Preferably, place carrier on floor If carrier is on table or other elevated surface, keep one hand on it Use restraint straps If you wear a soft carrier, bend from knees, not waist
Suffocation and positional asphyxia	birth to 8 months	Never place carrier on bed, couch, or other soft surface Position carrier at angle recommended by manufacturer Follow age and weight recommendations
Shopping carts		
Falls	2 years	Place child in seat and use restraint straps Do not allow children to ride or hang on outside of cart Do not allow children in cart's basket

*Children outside these age ranges can also suffer these kinds of injuries, but children in the age range given suffer them most often.

CHART 6
HOUSEHOLD ENVIRONMENT

Injury	Age at Highest Risk*	How to Prevent Injury
Allergies and respiratory problems related to poor air quality	all ages	Replace filters in heating and air conditioning systems regularly Install carbon monoxide detector Refrain from smoking Have vented heating systems checked yearly Dust, mop, and vacuum regularly
Falls		
Down stairs	1 to 2 years	Use baby gates at top and bottom of stairs Keep doors to basement and other stairs closed and locked
From windows	1 to 5 years	Limit children's access to windows: do not put furniture that children can climb onto near windows; do not position crib or bed next to window Use window guards (screen alone will not keep a child from falling out window)
Lead poisoning	all ages	If you live in an older house, have a professional inspect for lead paint If you have lead pipes, run water for a few minutes before using it for the first time each day Avoid leaded miniblinds If you suspect lead poisoning, have children's blood checked for lead
House fires		
General precautions	all ages	Make sure smoke detectors are functioning Practice an evacuation drill Teach children to stop, drop, and roll Store flammables away from ignition sources

Continued

CHART 6 HOUSEHOLD ENVIRONMENT
Continued

Injury	Age at Highest Risk*	How to Prevent Injury
From candles	all ages	Do not leave lit candles unattended When leaving room, blow out candles Do not place lit candles near bedding, drapes, or other flammable materials
From child play	all ages	Keep matches, cigarette lighters, and multipurpose lighters away from children
From gasoline and other flammables	all ages	Do not store gasoline in your home Do not store gasoline-operated tools (for example, lawn mower) in your home unless they are empty of fuel Do not use flammable substances around open flames or pilot light of furnace or water heater
From electrical sources	all ages	Do not use extension cords unless necessary, and then use correct size and length Do not run electrical cords under rugs Check cords on all electrical appliances and stop using worn or frayed cords Unplug small appliances not in use Have an electrician inspect the home for compliance with current electrical codes
Gunshots	all ages	Avoid having a gun in the house, but if you must, store it unloaded, in a locked box, out of children's reach Keep ammunition locked and separate from gun
Backyard injuries		
With lawn care	2 to 5 years	Have children remain inside while lawn is being mowed and while other power yard tools are in use

CHART 6 HOUSEHOLD ENVIRONMENT
Continued

Injury	Age at Highest Risk*	How to Prevent Injury
		Be aware that ride-on mowers are especially dangerous, because operator cannot see a young child behind the mower Keep lawn chemicals in locked area Avoid poisonous plants
Drowning in pools	1 to 4 years	Pool should have locked gate or other mechanism that young children cannot operate alone Barrier should be 4 feet high and in good repair Remove toys and playthings from pool area when finished so children do not come back for them later Never leave children alone in pool area Keep a phone near you in case of emergency Learn CPR
Drowning in ponds and creeks	1 to 4 years	Avoid ponds and creeks, because it is difficult to set up a barrier between a child and the water Do not leave children alone in a backyard with pond or creek Learn CPR
Drowning in five-gallon and other buckets	12 to 20 months	Empty buckets of liquids as soon as you finish cleaning task Do not store buckets where they can collect rain Learn CPR

*Children outside these age ranges can also suffer these kinds of injuries, but children in the age range given suffer them most often.

Chart 7
ROOM BY ROOM

Injury	Age at Highest Risk*	How to Prevent Injury
Kitchen		
Mechanical injury	1 to 5 years	Store knives and other sharp items out of child's reach After use, unplug appliances, like blenders, that have cutting blades Keep trash cans covered—discarded broken glass often causes cuts Make sure stove is secured to prevent tip-over
Thermal injury: contact burn	1 to 2 years	Keep child confined in high chair, playpen, or other enclosed space so he cannot reach hot surfaces
Thermal injury: scald burn	1 to 2 years	Keep child confined in high chair, playpen, or other enclosed space so she cannot reach hot liquids Use back burners on stove, if possible Turn pot handles toward back of stove Keep coffeepots, deep fryers, and other appliances at rear of counter, out of child's reach Do not let appliance cords dangle off counter Do not use tablecloths or placemats Do not carry child while you are cooking Do not have child sit on your lap while you eat or drink hot foods or liquids
Electrical injury: shock	(uncommon in kitchens)	Unplug electric appliances when not in use
Chemical injury: burn and poisoning	1 to 3 years	Lock accessible cabinets where chemicals (cleaners, bleaches, drain solvents, etc.) are kept Keep products in their original, labeled containers Keep handy the phone number for poison control; the National Poison Control Hotline is 1-800-222-1222

CHART 7 ROOM BY ROOM
Continued

Injury	Age at Highest Risk*	How to Prevent Injury
Living or family room		
Falls onto furniture	1 to 3 years	Install protective caps on corners of furniture, especially coffee table Install barrier around fireplace, wood-stove
Furniture tip-over	1 to 4 years	Make sure TV is on stable surface, preferably out of child's reach Securely attach bookcases and shelving to wall Avoid pedestal tables, which can tip easily
Suffocation in pillows	birth to 12 months	Do not put baby to sleep on sofa or soft chair Do not put baby in carrier on top of sofa or soft chair
Electric shock	1 to 3 years	Cover electrical outlets with safety plugs
Bedroom		
Suffocation in bed	3 to 6 months	Do not take infant into your bed to sleep the entire night: the most common cause of infant suffocation is wedging between bed and wall, no matter how close bed is to wall Do not put baby in carrier on top of bed Do not put baby to sleep on water bed
Suffocation in storage areas	1 to 4 years	Lock hope chests and similar furniture
Furniture tip-over	1 to 4 years	Put heavier items in bottom drawers to stabilize furniture
Poisoning	1 to 3 years	Store medicines out of child's reach

Continued

CHART 7 ROOM BY ROOM
Continued

Injury	Age at Highest Risk*	How to Prevent Injury
Bathroom		
Drowning	5 months to 2 years	Never leave children alone in bathtub, even if you use a bath ring or bath seat Close and lock toilet lid Never entrust young child to slightly older sibling
Scald burn	1 to 2 years	Never leave children alone in the bath Seat child to face opposite faucet Never entrust young child to slightly older sibling
Poisoning	1 to 3 years	Store prescription medicines, over-the-counter medicines, baby oil, and cosmetics out of child's reach
Laundry room		
Poisoning	1 to 3 years	Store bleach and detergents out of child's reach
Falls	birth to 5 years	Do not place infant in carrier on top of washer or dryer Do not let children climb onto washer or dryer
Shed, basement, garage, and other storage areas		
All injuries	birth to 5 years	Keep door to storage areas locked
Exercise room		
Friction burn	15 months to 3 years	Do not use treadmill or other equipment with moving parts when children are nearby Keep workout area off limits to children

*Children outside these age ranges can also suffer these kinds of injuries, but children in the age range given suffer them most often.

Resources

The following are sources of helpful injury prevention information. This is by no means an exhaustive list. New information is constantly being generated, so parents need to remain active in obtaining—and contributing—updated information. For example, the Consumer Product Safety Commission website makes it easy for anyone to file a complaint on line, as well as to find out about product recalls.

American Foundation for the Blind
    11 Penn Plaza, Suite 300
    New York, NY 10001
    800-232-5463
    www.afb.org

Boundless Playground National Resource Center
    968 Farmington Avenue
    West Hartford, CT 06117
    860-586-8990
    www.boundlessplaygrounds.org

Consumer Federation of America (CFA)
    1424 16th Street NW, Suite 604
    Washington, DC 20036
    202-387-6121
    www.consumerfed.org

Consumer Product Safety Commission
    Washington, DC 20207
    800-638-CPSC
    www.cpsc.gov

Consumers Union
    www.consumersunion.org

Food and Drug Administration
    www.fda.gov

Government recalls
    www.recalls.gov

Harborview Injury Prevention and Research Center
   http://depts.washington.edu/hiprc

Injury Free Coalition for Kids
   www.injuryfree.org

Kids In Danger
   116 W. Illinois, Suite 5E
   Chicago, IL 60610-4522
   312-595-0649
   Fax 312-595-0939
   www.kidsindanger.org

National Center for Injury Prevention and Control
   www.cdc.gov/ncipc

National Fire Protection Association
   www.nfpa.org

National Highway Traffic Safety Administration
   www.nhtsa.dot.gov

National Home Safety Council
   www.homesafetycouncil.org

National Playground Safety Institute (within the National Recreation
and Park Association)
   www.nrpa.org (scroll down list of Hot Topics to find National
   Playground Safety Institute)

National Program for Playground Safety
   School of Health, Physical Education, and Leisure Services
   University of Northern Iowa
   Cedar Falls, IA 50614
   319-273-2416
   www.uni.edu/playground

National Recreation and Park Association
   22377 Belmont Ridge Road
   Ashburn, VA 21048
   703-858-0784
   www.nrpa.org

New Parents Network
   www.npn.org

Nick Jr. Parenting
    www.nickjr.com/parenting/index.jhtml

Playground Industry Reference Directory
    800-352-1137
    www.world-playground.com

Safe Kids Worldwide
    1301 Pennsylvania Avenue NW, Suite 1000
    Washington, DC 20004–1707
    www.safekids.org

Toy Industry Foundation, Inc.
    1115 Broadway, Suite 400
    New York, NY 10010
    212-675-1141
    www.toy-tia.org

United States Access Board (access for the disabled to playgrounds,
among other things)
    www.access-board.gov

Bibliography

The information in this book is based on the relevant sections of the Code of Federal Regulations, relevant industry (ASTM) standards, and relevant materials from the U.S. Consumer Product Safety Commission and SAFE KIDS Worldwide. ("ASTM" refers to a standards development organization formerly known as American Society for Testing and Materials but now known simply as ASTM.) In addition, I based the text on my own experience and education and consulted the materials listed below.

Adler P. Injury data related to grocery/shopping carts. [memo]. Washington, DC: Consumer Product Safety Commission, November 18, 1994.

American Academy of Pediatrics (AAP). Car safety seats: a guide for families. Elk Grove Village, IL: The Academy, 2005.

———. First aid: choking/CPR. [poster]. Elk Grove Village, IL: The Academy, 2006.

———. Foods and choking in children. [conference report]. Evanston, IL: The Academy, 1983.

Andazola JJ, Sapien RE. The choking child: what happens before the ambulance arrives? Prehospital Emergency Care 1999 jan-mar;3(1):7–10.

Banever GT, Moriarty KP, Sachs BF, Courtney RA, Konefal SH, Barbeau L. Pediatric hand treadmill injuries. Journal of Craniofacial Surgery 2003 jul;14(4):487–90.

Barron's Educational Series. Atlas of anatomy. Hauppauge, NY: Barron's Educational Series, Inc., 1997.

Bluestone CD, Stool SE, editors. Pediatric otolaryngology. Philadelphia: W. B. Saunders, 1983.

Bolton D, Taylor BJ, Campbell AJ, Galland BC, Cresswell C. Rebreathing expired gases from bedding: a cause of cot death? Archives of Disease in Childhood 1993;69(2):187–90.

Bremner JG. Infancy. Second Ed. Oxford: Blackwell, 1994.

Citrin A, Leong G, Cuff D, Packer J, Butler L, Lester M. Let's play: a guide to toys for children with special needs. New York: Toy Industry Foundation, Inc., 2006.

Coalition for Consumer Health and Safety. Hidden hazards number one. Washington: The Coalition.

Consumer Product Safety Act (Public Law 92-573). October 27, 1972.

Consumer Product Safety Commission. CPSC, Graco Children's Products announce new safety instructions to prevent injuries with portable play yards. [press release]. Release 03-189. Washington, DC, 2003.

———. CPSC warns: Pools are not the only drowning danger at home for kids. [press release]. Release 02-169. Washington, DC, 2002.

———. Graco recalls cradle portion of swing based on reports of suffocation incidents. [press release]. Release 92-054. Washington, DC, 1992.

————. Recent death prompts search for recalled play yards/cribs. [press release]. Release 01-094. Washington, DC, 2003.

————. The safe nursery. Washington, DC: Consumer Product Safety Commission, 2000.

Cratty BJ. Perceptual and motor development in infants and children. Third Ed. Englewood Cliffs, NJ: Prentice-Hall, 1986.

Decina LE, Lococo KH. Child restraint system use and misuse in six states. Accident: Analysis and Prevention 2005;37(3):583–90.

Drago DA. Kitchen scalds and thermal burns in children five and younger. Pediatrics 2005;115(1):10–16.

Drago DA, Dannenberg AL. Infant mechanical suffocation in the United States, 1980–1997. Pediatrics 1999;103(5):e59.

Drago DA, Winston FK, Baker S. Clothing drawstring entrapment in playground slides and school buses: contributing factors and potential interventions. Archives of Pediatric and Adolescent Medicine 1997 jan;151:72–77.

Durbin DR, Chen I, Smith R, Elliott MR, Winston FK. Effects of seating position and appropriate restraint use on the risk of injury to children in motor vehicle crashes. Pediatrics 2005:115(3):e305.

Elder J. Safe sleeping for babies. Consumer Product Safety Review (Consumer Product Safety Commission) vol5 no1, summer 2000.

Federal Hazardous Substances Act (Public Law 86-613). July 12, 1960.

Flammable Fabrics Act (Public Law 83-88). June 30, 1953.

Food and Drug Administration, Office of Cosmetics and Colors. Sunscreens, tanning products, and sun safety. [fact sheet]. June 27, 2000.

Heimlich maneuver instructions. [website www.heimlichinstitute.org]. Cincinnati, OH: Heimlich Institute, 2005.

Henriques FC. Studies of thermal injury V: The predictability and the significance of thermally induced rate processes leading to irreversible epidermal injury. Archives of Pathology 1947;489–502.

Katcher ML. Tap water scald prevention: it's time for a worldwide effort. [editorial]. Injury Prevention 1998;4:167–9.

Kemp JS, Kowalski RM, Burch PM, Graham MA, Thach BT. Unintentional suffocation by rebreathing: a death scene and physiologic investigation of a possible cause of sudden infant death. Journal of Pediatrics 1993;122(6):874–80.

Kyle SB, Hayes J. Bean bag chairs. Consumer Product Safety Review (Consumer Product Safety Commission) vol12 no1, summer 1997.

Lawrenz AC, Fong D. Epidural haematoma and stroller-associated injury. Journal of Paediatrics and Child Health 1997;33(5):446–47.

Lawrenz K, Mayr JM, Seisser B. Shopping cart related accidents: are the preventive measures ineffective? International Journal of Injury Control and Safety Promotion 2000;7(3):195–204.

Maguina P, Palmieri TL, Greenhalgh DG. Treadmills: a preventable source of pediatric friction burn injuries. Journal of Burn Care and Rehabilitation 2004 mar-apr;25(2):201–4.

Moore L, Bayard R. Pathological findings in hanging and wedging deaths in infants and young children. American Journal of Forensic Medicine and Pathology 1993;14(4):296–302.

Moritz AR, Henriques FC. Studies of thermal injury II. The relative importance of time and surface temperature in the causation of cutaneous burns. American Journal of Pathology 1947;23:695–720.

National Center for Injury Prevention and Control. Injury Fact Book, 2001–2002. Atlanta: Centers for Disease Control and Prevention, 2001.

National Committee for Injury Prevention and Control. Injury Prevention: Meeting the Challenge. New York: Oxford University Press, 1989.

Poison Prevention Packaging Act (Public Law 91-601). December 3, 1970.

Pollack-Nelson C, Drago DA. Supervision of children aged two through six years. International Journal of Injury Control and Safety Promotion 2002;9(2):121–26.

Powell E, Jovtis E, Tanz R. Incidence and description of stroller-related injuries. Pediatrics 2002;110(5):e62.

Qureshi S, Mink R. Aspiration of fruit gel snacks. Pediatrics 2003 mar;111(3):687–89.

Rauchschwalbe R, Brenner RA, Smith GS. The role of bathtub seats and rings in infant drowning deaths. Pediatrics 1997;100(4):e1.

Rauchschwalbe R, Mann NC. Pediatric window-cord strangulations in the United States, 1981–1995. Journal of the American Medical Association 1997;277(21):1696–98.

Refrigerator Safety Act (Public Law 84-930). August 2, 1956.

Schneider D, Freeman N. Children's environmental health: reducing risk in a dangerous world. Washington, DC: American Public Health Association, 2000.

Seidel J, Gausche-Hill M. Lychee-flavored gel candies: a potentially lethal snack for infants and children. Archives of Pediatric and Adolescent Medicine 2002 nov;156(11):1120–22.

Simon HK, Tamura T, Colton K. Reported level of supervision of young children while in the bathtub. Ambulatory Pediatrics 2003;3(2):106–8.

Snyder RG, Schneider LW, Owings CL, Reynolds HM, Golomb DH, Schork MA. Anthropometry of infants, children, and youths to age 18 for product safety design. Report UM-HSRI-77-17. Washington, DC: Consumer Product Safety Commission, 1977.

Warr R, Drew P. Mummy's little helper. [letter to editor]. Burns 2002 sep;28(6):617.

White BL. The First Three Years of Life. Revised Ed. New York: Prentice-Hall, 1986.

Index